THE AGING LUMBAR SPINE

SAM W. WIESEL, M.D.

Department of Orthopaedic Surgery
George Washington University
School of Medicine
Washington, D.C.

PHILLIP BERNINI, M.D.

Section of Orthopaedic Surgery
Dartmouth-Hitchcock Medical Center
Assistant Clinical Professor of Orthopaedic Surgery
Dartmouth Medical School
Hanover, New Hampshire

RICHARD H. ROTHMAN, M.D., Ph.D.

Head, Section of Orthopedic Surgery
Pennsylvania Hospital
Philadelphia, Pennsylvania

1982
W. B. SAUNDERS COMPANY
Philadelphia   London   Toronto   Mexico City   Rio de Janeiro   Sydney   Tokyo

W. B. Saunders Company: West Washington Square
                           Philadelphia, PA   19105

                           1 St. Anne's Road
                           Eastbourne, East Sussex BN21 3UN, England

                           1 Goldthorne Avenue
                           Toronto, Ontario M8Z 5T9, Canada

                           Cedro 512
                           Mexico 4, D.F., Mexico

                           Rua Coronel Cabrita, 8
                           Sao Cristovao Caixa Postal 21176
                           Rio de Janeiro, Brazil

                           9 Waltham Street
                           Artarmon, N.S.W. 2064, Australia

                           Ichibancho, Central Bldg., 22-1
                           Chiyoda-ku, Tokyo 102, Japan

Library of Congress Cataloging in Publication Data

Wiesel, Samuel.

The aging lumbar spine.

1. Spine – Surgery.   2. Spine – Aging.   3. Spine –
   Diseases.   4. Spine – Abnormalities.   I. Bernini,
   Phillip.   II. Rothman, Richard H., 1936–   .
   III. Title. [DNLM: 1. Lumbar vertebrae.   2. Lumbosacral
   region.   3. Spinal diseases – In old age. WE 750 W651a]

RD533.W53   618.97'673   81–40678

ISBN 0–7216–9336–9   AACR2

The Aging Lumbar Spine   ISBN   0-7216-9336-9

Last digit is the print number: 9   8   7   6   5   4   3   2   1

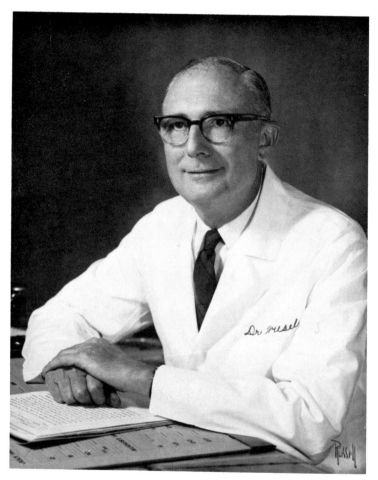

*We wish to respectfully dedicate this effort to our
teachers, as exemplified by Dr. Bert H. Wiesel.*

PREFACE

The population of people over the age of 60 is growing at a rapid rate. The lumbar spine in this group is universally affected by some degree of degenerative change, and thus the complaint of low back pain is common. In the past, these patients were told that nothing could be done for their back pain and that they should simply decrease their activity level. Many lived out their lives in a rocking chair as "spectators" to daily activities. Today, however, with the emphasis on physical fitness and modern advances in systemic care of the aged, the uniform prescription of decreased activity level is not well accepted.

The purpose of this monograph is to isolate the problems of the aging lumbar spine and present a current clinical approach to diagnosis and treatment. The majority of elderly patients can in fact be significantly improved, and certainly the majority should be able to function as active citizens in daily life.

The topics included here are those that primarily affect the aging lumbar spine and should be included in a differential diagnosis of low back pain in the older patient. By far the most common problem is osteoarthritis, and the pathophysiology of this subject is presented in depth.

It is hoped that after reading this monograph, the physician will be able to take an organized clinical approach to the elderly patient with back pain. It will also be appreciated that there are many questions yet to be resolved. This monograph is an initial attempt to deal with this increasingly important group of patients.

CONTENTS

Chapter 1

DEVELOPMENTAL ANATOMY AND PATHOPHYSIOLOGY OF LUMBAR DISC DISEASE

GENERAL INTRODUCTION

Pathologic conditions can be appreciated and better understood if one can grasp the natural history of the specific organ system that is involved. The lumbar spine in man is subject to an aging phenomenon that, if not understood, can precipitate erroneous cause-and-effect interpretation in the clinical setting, which might lead to unnecessary or inappropriate treatment regimens.

The goal of this chapter is to trace the development and growth of the spine and the natural aging phenomenon that affects the lumbar spine and the intervertebral disc in particular. We do not aim to provide a comprehensive discussion of all aspects of growth and development but rather those features that have practical significance in the appreciation of all aspects of lumbar spine disease.

At the outset, one must realize that any structure that contributes to the functional stability and integrity of the lumbar spine can contribute to its functional disability when that structure is compromised by disease or weakened by the biochemical and biomechanical changes that occur naturally with time. Moreover, as a result of the intimate functional relationships of these various structures, the relatively uninvolved components are overtaxed when the structures that are more affected by disease or aging are unable to realize their full supportive responsibilities. Although these structural components themselves can be the nidus of a pain problem, the secondary changes will frequently compromise the susceptible neurovascular elements of the lumbar spine. Therefore, a discussion of the components of the spine is an appropriate preface to a delineation of the clinical syndromes of the aging lumbar spine.

EMBRYOLOGIC DEVELOPMENT

A brief review of the basic embryologic development of the lumbar spine is a fitting introduction to the various functional components of the

1

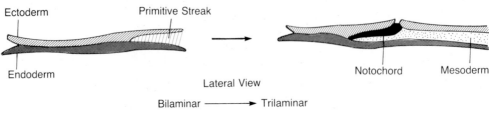

Figure 1–1. A bilaminar embryo.

axial skeleton that contribute to the clinical syndromes of lumbar disc "disease." Furthermore, such a review will shed light on the relatively common anomalies found in the spine as well as on those "normal variants" that may or may not have any pathologic significance. A more detailed review is provided by Ogden.[38]

During the second week of gestation, the embryo is a bilaminar disc composed of ectoderm and endoderm. At the beginning of the third week, an aggregation of cells termed the "primitive streak" develops within the ectoderm lamina. These cells localize between the ectoderm and the endoderm, forming the incipient mesoderm and subsequently the trilaminar embryo (Fig. 1–1).

This primitive streak, which is located in the midline of the embryonic disc, eventually generates the notochord, which in conjunction with the mesoderm will evolve into the many structural and functionally significant components of the axial skeleton. These notochord/mesodermal cells elongate in a cranial-caudal sequence and separate from the ectoderm and endoderm as the notochord eventually becomes tubular. Next, in an as yet unknown way, the cells induce the overlying ectoderm to form another aggregate of specialized cells known as the neural plate (Fig. 1–2). The notochord is an induction fulcrum of the axial skeleton which, if unaffected by teratogenic agents, has several functions. First, it will dissociate itself from the primtive gut or endoderm (excalation), thus preventing anomalous deformities between the axial skeleton and the intestinal cavity. Secondly, further ectodermal specialization is induced by the neural plate,

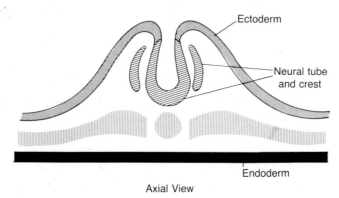

Figure 1–2. Axial view, trilaminar embryo.

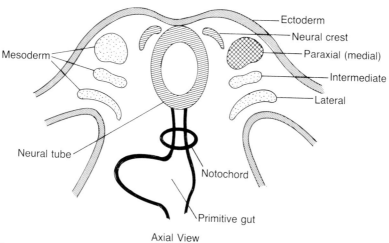

Axial View

Figure 1-3. Axial view, trilaminar embryo with subdivision of the primitive mesoderm into the medial paraxial, intermediate, and lateral columns.

leading to the formation of the neural tube, which when joined with the neural crest will become the central nervous system. Finally, the neural plate directs the medial paraxial column of the mesoderm to form the musculoskeletal components of the axial skeleton. It is uncertain whether the notochord directly dictates the mesodermal protection around the neural elements or whether it induces the neural elements to stimulate contiguous growth of the mesodermal components around itself (Fig. 1-3).

Clinically, a failure of the endoderm-notochordal dissociation can explain persistent neuroenteric canal deformities that are associated with numerous ventral vertebral body deformities (congenital scoliosis and kyphosis) (Fig. 1-4) and diastematomyelia (a diastasis of the spinal cord from bone, cartilage, or fibrous tissue that persists across the spinal canal in the sagittal plane) (Fig. 1-5). Induction deficiencies involving the ectodermal lamina can cause an obvious myelomeningocele with exposed matted nerves or a subtle dorsal sinus with or without a small hairy skin patch. Since the induction role of the notochord affects all three aspects of the trilaminar embryo, it would not be surprising to have deformities involving the structural components and the neurovascular components simultaneously. Finally, because the neural tube forms within the central aspect of the embryo and propagates cranial as well as caudal, the base of the spine will frequently be the site of developmental anomalies such as myelomeningocele or the frequently encountered spina bifida occulta (Fig. 1-6).

Toward the end of the third week of gestation, the paraxial columns of the mesoderm differentiate into the specific structural components of the spine, with the formation of somites in paired segments in a cranial (or rostral) to caudal direction (Fig. 1-7). Additionally, the paraxial columns give rise to (1) the outer skin and subcutaneous tissue of the axial skeleton known as the dermatome (Fig. 1-8), (2) a dorsal interlaminar aggregation

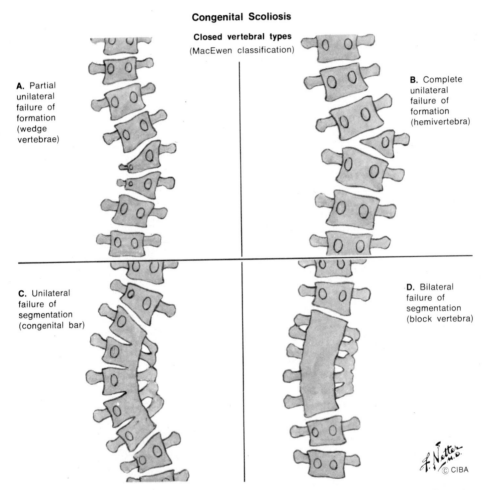

Congenital Scoliosis

Closed vertebral types
(MacEwen classification)

A. Partial
unilateral
failure of
formation
(wedge
vertebrae)

B. Complete
unilateral
failure of
formation
(hemivertebra)

C. Unilateral
failure of
segmentation
(congenital bar)

D. Bilateral
failure of
segmentation
(block vertebra)

Figure 1–4. McEwen classification, congenital scoliosis. Closed vertebra and extravertebral types. (© Copyright 1972 CIBA Pharmaceutical Company, Division of CIBA-GEIGY Corporation. Reproduced, with permission, from CIBA Clinical Symposium, *24*:1, 1972. All rights reserved.)

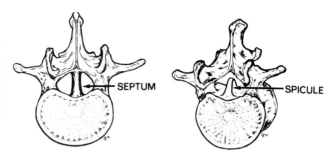

Figure 1–5. Diastematomyelia, which is the dichotomy of the spinal cord caused by either bone, cartilage, or fibrous tissue traversing the spinal canal in the sagittal plane. (From Hood, R. W., et al.: Diastomyelia and structural spinal deformities. J. Bone Joint Surg., 62*A*:520, 1980.)

of cells that contributes to the muscular and tendinous structures of the spine, and (3) the ventral inner layer (sclerotome) that becomes the osteocartilaginous skeleton.

This structural component development occurs with neural maturation, and a one somite–one neural component relationship is established early. It persists regardless of the occurrence of mesodermal migration and consequently explains the complex but well-defined problem of referred

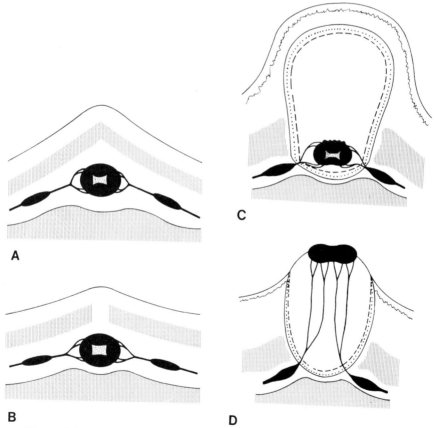

Figure 1–6. Four axial views of the spine. *A,* A normal spinal arrangement. *B,* A simple spina bifida occulta. *C,* A simple myelocele. *D,* Severe meningomyelocele. The spectrum of presentation depends upon the severity of the anomalous development of the lumbar spine.

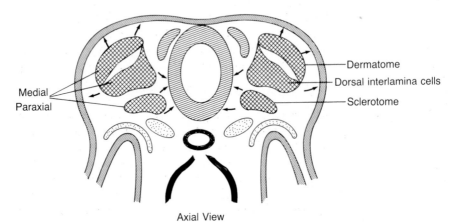

Axial View

Figure 1–7. Axial view, trilaminar embryo, with the medial paraxial columns giving rise to dermatome, dorsal interlaminar cells, and the sclerotome.

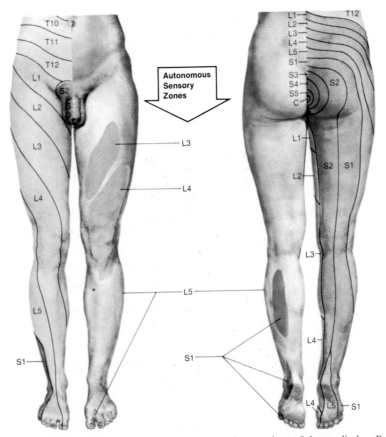

Figure 1–8. Dermatomes. Segmental sensory innervation of lower limbs. Pain is appreciated in these areas depending upon the specific spinal nerve root involved subsequent to the dermatome differentiation from the medial paraxial columns of the embryonic mesoderm. (© Copyright 1957, 1964 CIBA Pharmaceutical Company, Division of CIBA-GEIGY Corporation. Reproduced, with permission, from The CIBA Collection of Medical Illustrations by Frank H. Netter, M.D. All rights reserved.)

scrotal and inguinal pain that accompanies renal parenchymal disease (renal development originating in the intermediate column of the mesoderm) or the buttock and thigh pain (usually proximal) and occasional distal leg complaints that are associated with non-specific lumbosacral symptoms.[20, 28]

The sclerotome differentiates into cranial and caudal halves along a fissure known as the sclerotome fissure of von Ebner, allowing for bisegmental development of each vertebral motion segment (the vertebral body and the intervertebral disc) and subsequently for neurovascular involvement at two segments simultaneously (Fig. 1–9). The neural tube and crest provide the neurologic substrate around which mesenchymal structures are arranged, whereas paired segmental branches from the dorsal aorta or paired dorsal arteries provide the vascular components. It is critical that the clinician be aware of the clinical implications of this developmental sequence in the attempt to specifically identify a nidus of pain in the lumbar spine by pain pathways that are more often shared than individual.

Concomitantly with sclerotome differentiations (also known as resegmentation), the notochord becomes encased within the mesodermal lamina tissue, directly inducing anterior development of the spinal canal (the

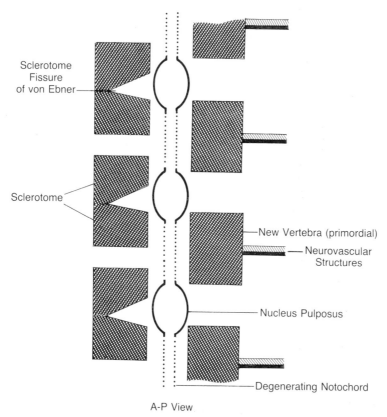

Sclerotome
Fissure
of von Ebner

Sclerotome

New Vertebra (primordial)

Neurovascular
Structures

Nucleus Pulposus

Degenerating Notochord

A-P View

Figure 1–9. Anteroposterior view of the lumbar spine with sclerotome differentiation occurring on the left about the sclerotome fissure of von Ebner with resegmentation recurring on the right.

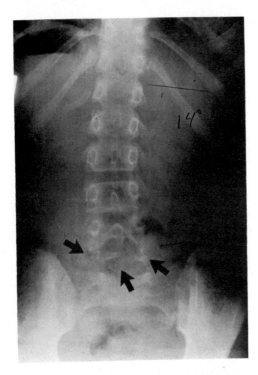

Figure 1–10. AP view of a child with spondylolisthesis demonstrating facet trophisms as well as spina bifida occulta. This patient had a type I spondylolisthesis (see classification chart).

vertebral bodies). The notochord probably indirectly induces posterior development (the lamina, spinous process, and the foramina) by some neurogenic inducer in the neural tube.[40] The ability of the notochord to induce development both directly and indirectly can therefore explain the occurrence of isolated anterior anomalies (failure of segmentation: vertebral bars and blocked vertebra; failure of formation: hemivertebra resulting from notochord induction deficiency as well as posterior anomalies (facet trophisms, spina bifida occulta, and even type I spondylolisthesis) caused by neural tube induction deficiencies (Fig. 1–10).

The defects in meningocele (neural elements protected by intact dura from the mesoderm) and myelomeningocele (neural elements exposed and unprotected) always occur in the posterior element, but a simple midline defect known as spina bifida occulta, found in up to 20 per cent of the general population and up to 30 per cent of the population with spondylolisthesis, is not associated with a neural defect.

The encased notochord that becomes trapped with the consolidating scleroderm (resegmentation) eventually degenerates. That segment between the individually developing incipient vertebra, derived from paraxial column tissue, becomes the substrate for the nucleus pulposus, which is encased by the annulus fibrosus. The presence of channel remnants of the notochord within the vertebral bodies and the end-plates may explain the origin of Schmorl's nodes, which develop under the physiologic pressures resulting from nucleus pulposus material herniating into the less substantial trabecula of the vertebral body (Fig. 1–11). Persistence of notochordal tissue that has not undergone mucoid degeneration may be an explanation for the manifestation of the neoplasm chordoma, with its characteristic

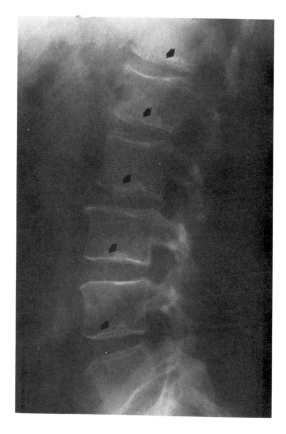

Figure 1–11. Lateral x-ray of the spine showing a Schmorl's node with nuclear material herniating into the less substantial trabecula of the vertebral body. (From Rothman, R. H., and Simeone, F. A.: The Spine, 2nd ed. Philadelphia, W. B. Saunders Co., 1982.)

mucoid-containing physaliphorous cells that are usually found at the rostral or caudal ends of the axial skeleton. This segmental development occurs within the fourth to sixth week of gestation, after which time chondrofication begins.

CHONDRO-OSSIFICATION

The vertebrae are the components of the spine that protect the neurovascular structures and provide moorings for the multiple muscles and ligaments that permit motor function and stabilize the spine. The conversion of embryonic tissue to chondral and then osseous tissue is a slow but deliberate process. With skeletal maturation, the osteochondral tissue continues to change as the spine accommodates the increasing forces and adverse effects of aging. Chondro-ossification is only the first step in a life-long dynamic process affecting the lumbar vertebrae.

The lumbar vertebra is produced by two anterior, two posterior, and two lateral centers of chondrofication. Concomitantly, the annulus is derived from the perichondrial ring at the scleroderm fissure of von Ebner; therefore, all but the nucleus pulposus are of mesodermal origin. Ossification of the primary centers within the vertebral bodies begins in the fourth month of gestation, and by the fifth to the sixth month, the

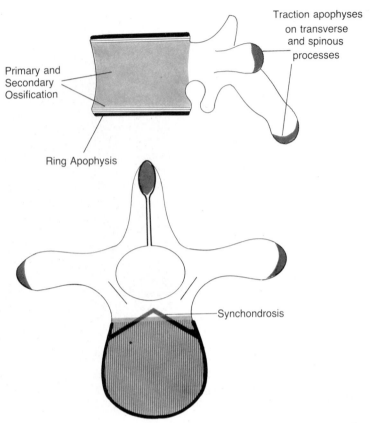

Figure 1–12. Primary and secondary centers of ossification and traction apophyses. Also noted is the vertebral synchondrosis.

epiphyseal plates at the cranial and caudal ends of each vertebra begin to ossify. The ring apophyses, which are secondary ossification centers that attach the annulus to the vertebral body end-plate, do not begin to ossify until the second decade of life and may not unite with the parent vertebral body until the end of the third decade of life. This unification is the ultimate sign of axial skeletal maturation (Fig. 1–12).

The primary ossification centers of the vertebral bodies and the posterior elements occur in the plane anterior to the pedicle (the anatomic connection of the anterior and posterior elements). This site, referred to as the neurocentral synchondrosis, is not to be confused with either the pedicle or the pars interarticularis (the part between the articular surfaces of the facets) (Fig. 1–13) and is not responsible for the typical spondylolytic lesion (type II A or type II B spondylolisthesis), which is more likely a result of stress fractures than developmental or congenital lesions (see Table 9–9).[46]

Faulty closure of the synchrondrosis, however, can change the sagittal dimensions of the spinal canal and contribute to the development of congenital anomalies involved in spinal stenosis (Table 1–1),[3] which is especially marked in persons with achondroplasia, who develop varying

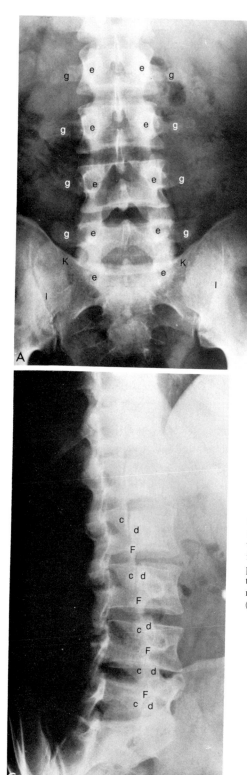

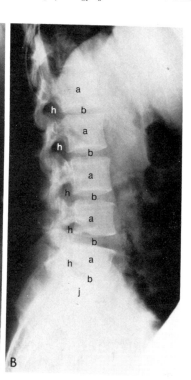

Figure 1–13. *A*, AP, *B*, lateral, and *C*, oblique x-rays of a normal lumbar spine with anatomy labeled: (a) lumbar vertebra; (b) intervertebral disc; (c) inferior facet; (d) the superior facet; (e) the pedicle; (F) the pars interarticularis; (g) transverse process; (h) the neural foramina; (I) sacroiliac joint; (j) sacrum; and (k) sacral ala.

TABLE 1–1. Classification of the Spinal Configurations Contributing to Lumbar Spinal Stenosis and Nerve Root Entrapment Syndromes.[3]

1. Congenital – Developmental Stenosis
   a) Idiopathic
   b) Achondroplastic
2. Acquired Stenosis
   a) Degenerative
      i) Central Portion of Spinal Canal
      ii) Peripheral Portion of Canal, Lateral Recesses, and Nerve Root Canals (tunnels).
      iii) Degenerative Spondylolisthesis
   b) Combined
      Any possible combinations of congenital/developmental stenosis, degenerative stenosis, and herniations of the nucleus pulposus.
   c) Spondylolisthetic/Spondylolytic
   d) Iatrogenic
      i) Post laminectomy
      ii) Post fusion (anterior and posterior)
      iii) Post chemonucleolysis
   e) Post-Traumatic, late changes
   f) Miscellaneous
      i) Paget's Disease
      ii) Fluorosis

manifestations of acute or intermittent neurogenic claudication (Fig. 1–14). In most cases, however, the varying amounts of space available for the neural elements, which can be determined by noninvasive ultrasound techniques and computerized axial tomography, are manifestations of the time range within which the fusion of these primary ossification centers can

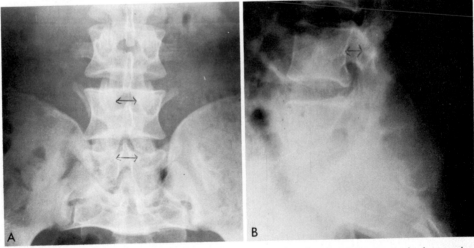

Figure 1–14. *A,* AP and *B,* lateral x-ray of an achondroplast showing the compromised coronal and sagittal planes due to faulty closure of the synchondroses.

occur. One will encounter a varying three-dimensional spectrum of gross anatomic presentations as the spine is altered by age and postural change.

The inferior and superior facets that develop out of the sclerotome matrix are diarthrodial (synovial joints). These facets are affected by resegmentation, which means that the inferior and superior facets of two adjacent vertebrae at one time originated from different sclerotomes before resegmentation produced the individual intact vertebra. The completely formed lumbar vertebra is massive, providing a needed structural integrity for activity and protection for susceptible neurovascular elements. The initial sagittal orientation of the lumbar vertebra facets leading to the coronal plane orientation at the lumbosacral junction limits rotation significantly in the upper lumbar spine, whereas there is approximately 10 to 15 degrees of rotation caudally. There is a total of approximately 90 degrees of sagittal flexion and a more limited and varying degree of coronal flexion.

NEUROGENIC DEVELOPMENT

The clinical syndromes of lumbar disc disease that are most amenable to surgical intervention are usually associated with an objective neurologic deficit. It is essential that the physician be aware of the neural pathways and the relationship of those pathways to neighboring structures in order to determine the appropriate diagnosis and treatment.

Growth of the spinal cord, which is derived from the neural tube, lags behind the longitudinal growth of the axial skeleton. There is a relative ascent of the conus at the tip of the spinal cord from the level of the fifth lumbar vertebra at the third month of gestation to the lower part of the second lumbar vertebra at birth, and finally, to its adult location at the upper border of L2 at five years of age (Figure 1–15).[4]

The dura is derived from mesenchyma or mesoderm, whereas the leptomeninges (the pia and the arachnoid) are produced from the ectoderm. If there are developmental defects in induction, it is possible to have two nerve roots and the encompassing leptomeninges surrounded by a common dural sheath, a phenomenon encountered in anomalous nerve root disorders[5] (Fig. 1–16).

The conus medullaris evolves into the cauda equina, which is composed of the lumbar and sacral nerve roots responsible for lower extremity and major pelvic visceral motor and sensory activity. At each level, the intravaginal components of the dorsal and ventral spinal roots contribute to the true spinal nerves outside the neural foramina and distal to the dorsal root ganglion coming from the dorsal spinal root (Fig. 1–17). Pathology in or about the foramina, which are composed of the pedicle, annulus of the intervertebral disc, part of the vertebral body, and the superior facet at each level, can compromise the afferent and efferent fibers that provide motor function and sensation to the dorsum of the spine as well as to the lower extremities.

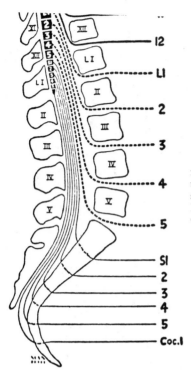

Figure 1–15. A lateral schematic of the spine showing the relationship of the conus to L1 and L2, and the relationship of the individual spinal nerves to each of the vertebral bodies at skeletal maturity. (From Haymaker, W., and Woodhall, B.: Peripheral Nerve Injuries, 2nd ed. Philadelphia, W. B. Saunders Company, 1953.)

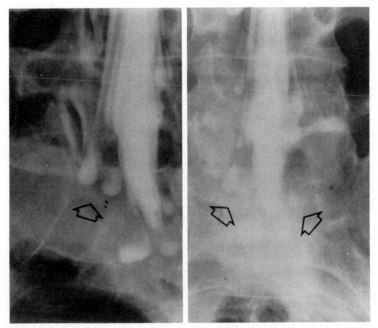

Figure 1–16. AP and oblique myelograms (metrizamide) of the lumbar spine demonstrating anomalous nerve roots: a conjoined nerve root exiting beneath the first sacral pedicle while no nerve root is exiting beneath the fifth pedicle.

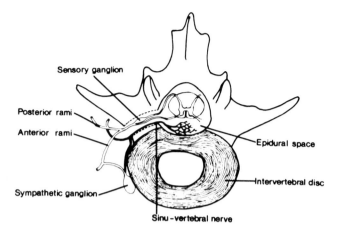

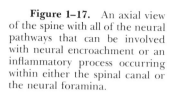

Figure 1–17. An axial view of the spine with all of the neural pathways that can be involved with neural encroachment or an inflammatory process occurring within either the spinal canal or the neural foramina.

Each lumbar nerve root exits below the pedicle of its accompanying vertebra. L4, L5, and S1 are the nerve roots that are affected in lumbar disc syndromes most often (99 per cent), but these, along with the lower sacral roots, can simultaneously be involved with various disease entities that can compromise all of the space that is available for the neural elements. The recurrent course of the sinu-vertebral nerve (see Fig. 1–17), coming from the posterior rami and also carrying sympathetic fibers, makes another afferent pathway that is susceptible to injury in a foramen compromised by injury, disease, or age. These characteristics make it extremely difficult to identify the *specific* component of the spine that has been injured, especially when there is no involvement of a well-defined nerve root.

VASCULAR ANATOMY

In the lumbar spine, the segmental lumbar arteries arising from the aorta supply both extraspinal and intraspinal structures, including the spinal medulla (the substance of the conus medullaris).[14] Blood is supplied to crucial intraspinal structures by way of the neural foramina, and the route is referred to as *radicular* when it provides blood to the nerve root exclusively, *medullary* if it supplies (in conjunction with the anterior and two posterior spinal arteries) the cord, and *spinal* if it distributes branches to the meninges, bone, and soft tissue of the axial skeleton (Fig. 1–18).[26, 39]

The intimate association of the vascular supply with the neural elements in both the spinal canal and the foramen is cause for speculation regarding the role of vascular compromise alone or in conjunction with neural compromise in the production of lumbar pain syndromes. Both probably occur simultaneously in varying degrees that cannot be quantified at this time (see Chapter Three.)

The venous supply to the lumbar spine mirrors the arterial supply. Batson[4] applied century-old knowledge of this system to various metastatic syndromes, but the relatively unique and consistent system has prompted the development of a diagnostic modality helpful in localizing mass lesions affecting the epidural space (Fig. 1–19) (see Chapter Two).

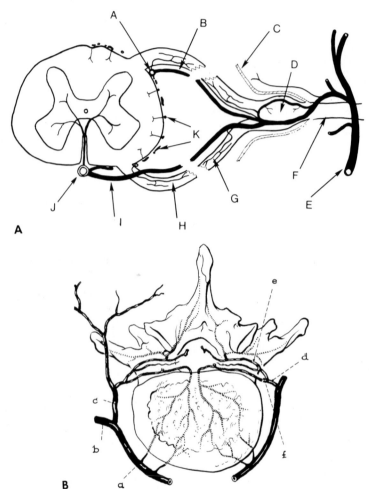

Figure 1–18. Arterial system of the lumbosacral spine. *A,* A schema illustrating all of the possible vascular relations of the spinal roots in which both medullary and radicular arteries are present. The break in the roots indicates that the schema applies to either the short cervical roots or the long lumbosacral elements of the cauda equina. The dorsolateral spinal artery (A) receives the dorsal medullary artery (B) and directly supplies the dorsal proximal radicular artery. The anterior spinal artery (J) receives the ventral medullary artery (I) and supplies the ventral proximal radicular artery (H) through the vasa corona (K). The segmental artery (E) gives a spinal branch that accompanies the spinal nerve (F) through the intervertebral foramen to supply the plexus of the dorsal root ganglion (D), which gives origin to the proximal radicular arteries (G) and (when present) the medullary vessels. The dura (C) receives fine meningeal branches. Note that medullary arteries usually do not supply roots in mid-course. (From Parke, W., Gammell, K., and Rothman, R.: Arterial vascularization of the cauda equina. J. Bone Joint Surg., *63A*:53, 1981.) *B,* Diagram of the blood supply to a vertebra as seen from below and from behind with the laminae removed. *a* is a segmental (in this case a lumbar) artery, *b* its ventral continuation, *c* its dorsal branch; *d* is the spinal branch, and *e* and *f* are the spinal branch's dorsal and ventral twigs to tissue of the epidural space and to the vertebral column; the unlabeled middle twig is to the nerve roots, and at some levels, to the spinal cord. (From Hollinshead, W. H.: Anatomy for Surgeons, Vol. 3. 2nd ed. New York, Harper and Row, 1969.)

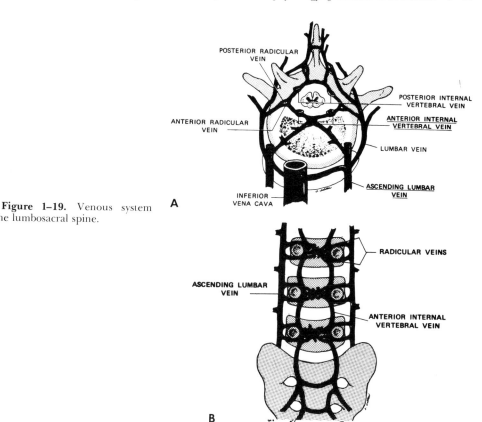

Figure 1–19. Venous system of the lumbosacral spine.

MUSCULOTENDINOUS COMPONENTS

As the neurovascular elements become surrounded by the axial cartilaginous and osseous skeleton, the simultaneously developing muscles and ligamentous complex developing from the paraxial column of the mesoderm span two or more levels, providing motion potential in three dimensions.

Overlying the spine, there are multisegmental muscles, which are usually superficial and are collectively called the sacrospinalis and transversospinalis, denoting origin, insertion, and course; the deeper unisegmental muscles are referred to as the segmental musculature.

All of these muscles are innervated by the posterior rami coming from the spinal nerves. It is crucial to realize that the posterior rami carry afferent pain fibers from the components of practically all of the structures (bone, muscle, ligaments, annulus, and facets) of the spine. Therefore, muscle spasm, which is appreciated so often clinically, is not necessarily a result of *direct* contusion or laceration (i.e., a primary pathologic state) but rather it may be a manifestation of some spinal reflex activity as a protective mechanism for some other injured or susceptible spinal component.

The anterior spinal musculature, namely, the quadratus lumborum and the iliopsoas, and the anterior musculature of the abdomen tend to cause flexion of the lumbar spine in the sagittal and coronal planes and, between them, antagonize the extensor forces of the dorsal musculature.

The dorsal muscles work dynamically to prevent a forward flexion motion of approximately 0 to 60 degrees from occurring; the complex posterior ligaments, referred to collectively as the posterior longitudinal system and made up of a complex interaction of supraspinous and intraspinous ligaments and lumbosacral fascia, statically support the spine after 60 degrees of forward flexion.[18] The dynamic and static support systems allow movement, maintain posture, and effectively dissipate energy that the spine is forced to absorb.

The intervertebral disc absorbs all forms of energy that are manifest as compression, shear, and tension and enables the facets, muscles, and ligaments to dissipate energy more gracefully. It is important to understand the pathophysiology of the lumbar disc and the anatomic, biochemical, and biomechanical changes that occur in this structure with aging. With this information, the natural aging process of the lumbar spine can be better understood, and the management of various disease states can be better formulated.

PATHOPHYSIOLOGY OF LUMBAR DISC DISEASE AND SPINAL STENOSIS

It is difficult to differentiate the pathophysiology of lumbar disc disease from the normal aging process that occurs primarily in the intervertebral disc and is reflected subsequently in the posterior elements. As clinicians, we deal with the clinical signs and symptoms of this aging process, but to consider the pathophysiology is to make no more than an assumption. This is particularly true since the changes seen in the spine grossly, roentgenographically, biomechanically, and biochemically affect all within a spectrum of presentation, any point within which symptoms may or may not arise.

Ontogenetic and Phylogenetic Changes

It may help to view aging and the pathophysiology of the lumbar spine ontogenetically as well as phylogenetically (Fig. 1–20 *A*). Phylogenetic changes give the lumbar spine pivotal importance in the progression from the quadriped status of the ape to the biped status of the human. One wonders if the development of the human lumbar spine is still lagging behind the functional demands of a biped orthograde stance, therefore making lumbar disc disease a temporary evolutionary flaw that will ultimately remedy itself within a millennium of aging while it paradoxically worsens within a few decades of human aging. Superimposed ontogenetic changes (Fig. 1–20 *B*) on the spine and the gradual evolution alluded to phylogenetically are reduced to mere decades as man is conceived, born, and ages. The condition is anatomically represented by the straight or

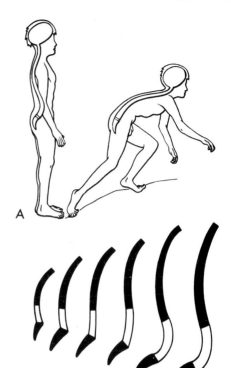

Figure 1–20. *A,* Phylogenic development. *B,* Ontogenic development.

kyphotic, minimally loaded spine of the neonate and the overloaded lordotic spine of the mature adult.

With the establishment of the lordotic posture of the lumbar spine, the adult configuration is reached, but the spine will insidiously and to varying degrees *age;* that aging will affect all components of the spine.

Changes Occurring with the Aging Process

In the first decades of life (Fig. 1–21), the gross appearance of the spine and its components will be basically unchanged. The intervertebral disc will maintain full height with a thickened, laminated annulus and a tense (preloaded) nucleus. The vertebrae are almost completely ossified, except for the apophyseal rings, and are nearly square in shape. The facets are well defined with smooth capsules and white-blue articular cartilage. The ligamentum flavum is only a few millimeters thick, and on the whole, the space that is available for the neural elements within the canal and the foramina is capacious and subsequently not encroached upon by any secondary changes in the many structural components. Some developmentally and congenitally narrowed spinal canals have much less space available in the first few decades of life, but symptoms are unusual.

In these first decades, one can anticipate finding asymptomatic disc

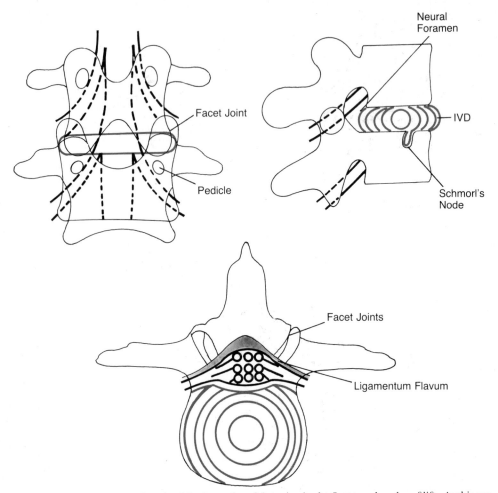

Figure 1–21. AP, lateral, and axial schematics of the spine in the first two decades of life. At this age, the neural structures can be compromised only by trauma, infection, neoplasm, and (relatively rare) posterior or posterolateral disc herniation.

herniations through the cartilaginous end-plate (Schmorl's nodes) and facet trophisms or asymmetric configurations in the development of the facets, but at this point in the aging process, these are not usually a well-defined source of pain or irritation; the possibility that they contribute to symptoms with further aging, however, can be postulated.

The third through the fifth decades of life show changes (Fig. 1–22) that can be quite pronounced, with the first manifestations of aging being reflected through the intervertebral disc. The biochemical changes (discussed in the following section) can produce one of three different phenomena: (1) degeneration of the annulus with disc nuclear herniation through the posterolateral annular rents, (2) nuclear degeneration with intact annulus, or (3) simultaneous degeneration of both the annulus and nucleus.[10] The biomechanical insufficiency of the involved disc compels the posterior elements, that is, the facets and capsules, to assume more compressive, tensile, and shear load, resulting in capsular strain, hypermobility, and articular cartilage fibrillation. This hypermobility can be manifest as traction spurs 1 to 2 mm. above the disc space anteriorly. The

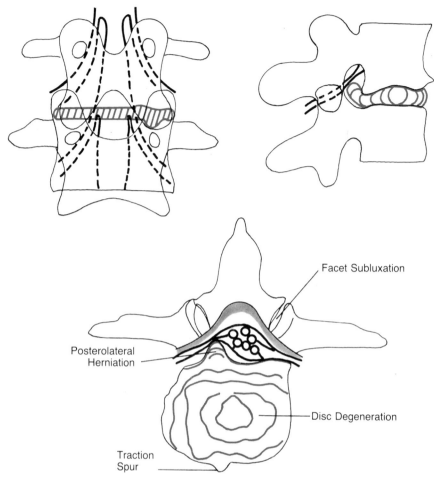

Figure 1–22. AP, lateral, and axial views of the spine, the third through the fifth decades, showing disc degeneration with herniation of the nuclear material. Facet joints in the axial view may show some subluxation, implying a hypermobile phase of motion segment instability. A typical traction spur is demonstrated on the lateral view.

ligamentum flavum will also be compelled to assume more tensile loads while becoming redundant as the total spine length decreases with disc degeneration. The vertebrae themselves tend toward a lowering and broadening in the superior, inferior, and midbody transverse breadth, a total change that, in static terms, begins to acutely or insidiously affect the neural elements.[16, 44]

If a disc herniation occurs in a spinal canal that is relatively small, compression of the neural elements will result, and a patient will experience symptoms. In pure terms, this can be thought of as a relative spinal stenosis. The stenosis occurs secondary to the herniated nucleus pulposus occupying space in a small spinal canal. On the other hand, a similar-sized disc herniation in a large spinal canal will cause no symptoms because the neural elements have enough room to escape pressure. Thus, symptoms in persons of this age group are a result not only of a disc herniation itself but are also dependent on the size of the spinal canal with which the individual is born.

Patients in the fourth decade of life and older (Fig. 1–23) can manifest

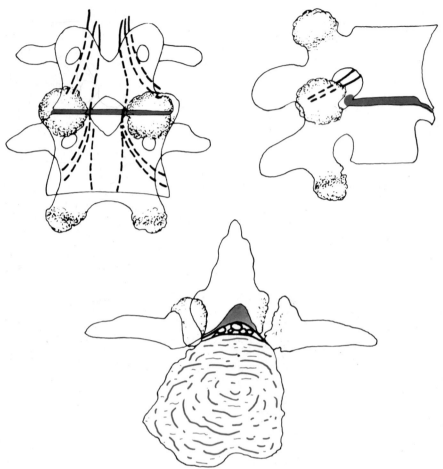

Figure 1–23. AP, lateral, and axial views of the fourth-decade-and-older spine show significant disc degeneration, a traction spur developing into a large osteophyte, and significant hypertrophic changes occurring within the facet joints compromising the neural elements both in the canal and in the neural foramina. Markedly thickened or redundant ligamentum flavum is also seen contributing to this neural compromise.

the hypomobile end-stage changes of the aging process. Degeneration of both facet joints and the intervertebral disc leads to a narrowing of the spinal canal. The canal is rimmed by large osteophytes, which develop in an effort to diminish the load on the now incompetent intervertebral disc. The facets are hypertrophic and deformed by osteophytic spurs that are encased within the thickened joint capsule. The ligamentum flavum becomes redundant and, in combination with the just-mentioned changes, the spinal canal and foramen are affected. Changes in the lumbar canal occur to some degree in all active people as they age. However, not everyone suffers from significant disability. The symptoms a person will have are dependent on the original size of the spinal canal. If the individual's spinal canal is small, the changes caused by aging in the disc and facet joints will lead to an absolute spinal stenosis with compression of the neural elements. If the spinal canal is large to begin with, the normal changes of aging will lead to a relative spinal stenosis with no neural compression.

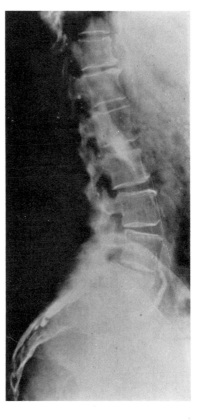

Figure 1–24. Spondylolisthesis resulting from degeneration occurring at L5–S1 with retrolisthesis occurring at L3–4. The direction of slip depends upon the location within the lumbar spine one is dealing with, but the slip itself is subsequent to both disc space degeneration and facet incompetence.

The previously discussed changes in the intervertebral disc and facet joints are associated with decreased movement in each motion segment. One may encounter either a retro- or a forward slip of one vertebral body on another owing to disc incompetence followed by facet subluxation. These slips are significant, but dynamic exaggeration is unusual (Fig. 1–24).

As the spine ages, one can also encounter postural alterations with a reduction in lordosis as the spine attempts to "decompress" the degenerating articular facets by maintaining a flexed rather than an extended posture. This flexed position can also provide more room for the susceptible neural elements within the canal and foramen, which are dynamically compromised in extension.

The decades of a person's life provide milestones within which most of the changes described will occur, but the overlap of these changes is extensive. It is essential to understand that the changes in no way dictate symptoms, define disability, or determine prognosis.

BIOCHEMICAL AND BIOMECHANICAL CHANGES IN THE INTERVERTEBRAL DISC

In practical and finite terms, if we examine the gross and radiographic changes in the lumbar spine structure as they relate to biochemical and subsequently biomechanical alterations in the intervertebral disc, we may still find it difficult to differentiate pathology from natural history. However, it may help to understand the various clinical syndromes that are associated with lumbar disc disease and subsequently determine a more rational treatment regimen for the symptoms.

A simple hypothesis that has guided research in the past two decades is that the biochemical alterations within the intervertebral disc contribute to structural insufficiency of the disc. This compels other structural components of the spine, namely, the facets and the joint capsules, to assume more responsibility. This relationship is eloquently described by Farfan as the "triple joint complex."[17] The concept of these biomechanical alterations has been elaborated on within the past decade by the suggestion that an autoimmune phenomenon in conjunction with the biochemical changes in the aging disc would propel the degenerative process and could coincidentally directly contribute to the development of various clinical syndromes.[35]

From the beginning, biomechanical changes have been correlated with poorly understood alterations in the nutrition of the intervertebral disc. As early as the late 1920s, it was proposed that the nutrition of the disc occurred through small blood vessels that reached the disc through the periphery of the annulus and across the cartilaginous end-plate. Unfortunately, the vessels begin to scar and dissipate as early as eight months of age and most probably by eight years of life.[41] With the exception of small peripheral annular vessels, the major blood supply to the disc, for all practical purposes, is gone by age 30. This phenomenon converts the minimally stressed vascular structure of infancy to a maximally stressed and relatively avascular structure by early middle age. The disc subsequently relies for nourishment upon the passage of nutrients and the elimination of waste products through the central portion of the cartilaginous end-plate and peripherally through the annulus. This may seem adequate at first, particularly if the vascular loss occurs insidiously over two decades; however, the disc nourishment is less than ideal if one considers the route by which the major nutrients enter the disc as well as the distribution of the various biochemical components that make up the intervertebral disc.

The nucleus pulposus, localized primarily at the junction of the middle and posterior third of the disc, is formed of a gelatinous and mucoid matrix within a loose (collagenous) fibrous strand network. There are some remaining notochordal cells initially, but they eventually vanish. The fluid content, which is approximately 90 per cent in the full term fetal disc, decreases to approximately 65 per cent in the geriatric adult intervertebral disc. The matrix is composed of interstitial fluid that primarily includes water and proteoglycan subunits. These subunits are noncollagenous protein cores with attached sulfated glucosaminoglycans of chondroitin-4 and chrondroitin-6 sulfate and keratan sulfate. These proteoglycan aggregates are attached to the long chains of hyaluronic acid by small glycoprotein links[8] (Fig. 1–25 *A, B*).

The collagen fibers are partly type II collagen, that is, the collagen that is found primarily in hyaline cartilage.[23] It should be remembered that the aging phenomenon that affects the matrix, specifically the proteoglycans and the fibrous collagen network of the intervertebral disc, will also affect

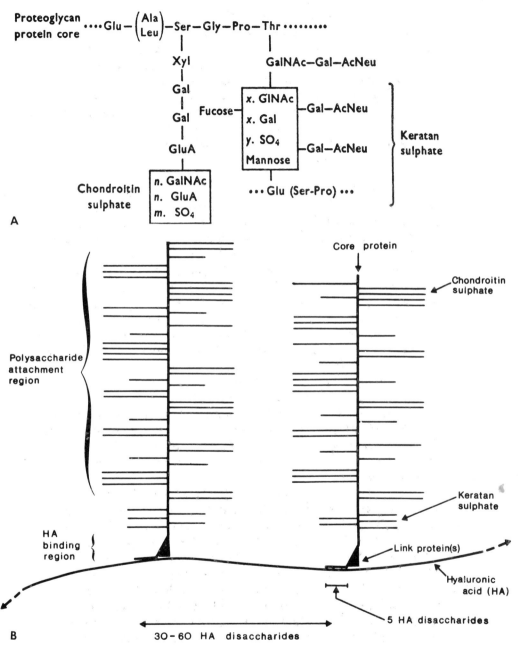

Figure 1–25. Composite of the glucosaminoglycans that make up proteoglycans, which, in turn, contribute to the much larger proteoglycan aggregates. *A,* Proposed structure for chondroitin sulphate–keratan sulphate–protein unit. (From Hopwood, J. J., and Robinson, H. C.: The structure and composition of cartilage keratan sulphate. Biochem. J. *141*:517, 1974.) *B,* Model of proteoglycan aggregation. (From Bushell, G. R., et al.: Proteoglycan chemistry of the intervertebral disks. Clin. Orthop., *129*:115, 1977.)

the same components in the neighboring end-plate and the facets of the triple joint complex. Aging is in parallel, although the clinical syndromes may be manifest in series.

The annulus fibrosus or the laminosis for the limiting membrane is composed primarily of type I collagen in the outermost regions and type II collagen closer to the nucleus.[2] It is of interest that the quadruped, e.g., the pig, has more type I collagen throughout, which presumably provides increased tensile strength, such as in tendons. Man, the biped, has more type II collagen that, like hyaline cartilage, must also resist compressive loads. This has been studied experimentally, and it has been demonstrated that the annulus, which is composed of a higher ratio of collagen to proteoglycan than is found in the nucleus pulposus, resists compressive loads and repeated loading quite well, even after discectomy (the removal of the nuclear center).[31] The compressive strength of the annulus as a result of type II collagen, in conjunction with the matrix, is impressive when one remembers that under excessive axial load, the vertebral body will fail before the annulus and the remainder of the intervertebral disc that has not been compromised by injury or by some type of degenerative or metabolic disease will fail.[30] The kangaroo, with its large and convenient tail, has a proportion of type I and type II collagen at some point between the collagen of the biped and the quadruped and, perhaps, has the best of both worlds regarding the matrix and fluid content of the annulus. The other components of the disc, the proteoglycan aggregate and water content, significantly diminish going from the central portion of the annulus to the periphery.

The distribution of proteoglycan and collagen is almost paradoxic, since the diffusion of the negatively charged solutes, such as sulfates, which is so essential for the turnover of the proteoglycans that are located primarily in the annulus, occurs mainly through the annulus fibrosus (the anterior more than the posterior aspect) and not through the end-plate directly into the nucleus, where the proteoglycans are primarily accumulated.[43] The diffusion of small, uncharged solutes such as glucose, occurs mainly through the end-plates and not through the annulus, where most of the collagen is localized. To add insult to injury, the posterior aspect of the annulus in the lumbar spine has a smaller surface area for diffusion of nourishment and is under greater strain than is the anterior aspect of the disc, and both the matrix and fiber content have a very slow metabolic turnover (over 500 days for the proteoglycans and even longer for the collagen); this makes not only maintenance but repair a significant task. Compound this inadequate nutrient delivery system with the decrease in the permeability of the disc material matrix that occurs with age,[7] and aging looks more and more pathologic.

If the cartilage end-plate is disrupted by vertebral loading and there are a diminished number of vascular contacts between the narrow space of the vertebral bodies and the degenerating hyaline cartilage of the end-plate, the nutrient delivery system can be rendered inadequate. In lumbar disc syndromes, the nutrient delivery system to the intervertebral disc is probably crucial. Although the disc is most likely the major route by which the spine can gracefully dissipate energy and enable the facets, muscles, ligaments, and bones to assume compressive shear and tensile loads, the production and maintenance of the proteoglycan aggregate with water and collagen is essential for proper intervertebral disc function. The nonlinear, viscoelastic quality of the intervertebral disc can in part be explained by the interaction of the proteoglycans, which have the ability to absorb energy, in compression with collagen, which has the ability to resist tensile loads as well as compression. The hoop stress energy dissipation[29] that is ideal in the young or minimally aged intervertebral disc is lost almost as soon as the biped stance is realized.

Under the load in the annulus, as well as in the nucleus pulposus, water is forced within the molecular structure of the glucosaminoglycans, chondroitin sulfate, and keratan sulfate on the proteoglycan aggregate. It has been suggested, however, that with aging and, presumably, with inadequate nutrition, proteoglycans are unable to form aggregates in the presence of hyaluronic acid. Although there is a relatively decreased water content, the inability of the nucleus pulposus particularly to imbibe water under load significantly decreases the ability of the disc to dissipate energy. The smaller proteoglycans and the relatively increased number of keratan sulfate glucosaminoglycans that have been found in degenerative discs are either inadequately synthesized or represent breakdown products of overload.[1, 23]

The proteoglycans have also become more mechanically integrated with the collagen with age and therefore lose their water-binding capabilities. At the same time, the entire dry weight percentage of the disc increases primarily because of a greater collagen content and a larger accumulation of noncollagenous proteins called "beta proteins," which can be identified by their unoriented x-ray fiber refraction patterns.[23, 25] These beta proteins may very well represent insoluble proteins resulting from collagen degeneration, which is a reasonable assumption in that, under electron microscopy, the collagen shows increased crystallinity precipitation and fibrillation. The collagens, therefore, fail to adequately resist tension and compression load as their nourishment is compromised by an inadequate delivery system.

The adverse alterations in the nutrient delivery system to the intervertebral disc probably result in undesirable biochemical changes and ultimately diminish the biomechanical efficiency of the intervertebral disc, forcing more load-dissipating responsibility on the other supporting components of the spine and producing clinical syndromes and roentgenographic changes that are familiar to all of us.

Indeed, if the annulus fails while the nucleus is still effectively imbibing water under load, disc herniation is possible. Under these circumstances, one may encounter the clinical syndrome of disabling back pain with or without well-defined, severe, lancinating sciatica, usually in the younger population. Nachemson's[34] work in in vivo intradiscal pressures (see Fig. 3–2) has received excellent clinical verification in that, in these younger individuals, one can correlate increasing pain in the low back, with or without leg pain, with increased intradiscal pressures, a phenomenon that is described often and is typified by the patient's reluctance to sit and stand and his preference for supine and side-lying positions because of pain aggravation. The accompanying x-ray of such a patient would most likely be unimpressive, which is not unexpected.

If the nucleus pulposus desiccates before the annulus loses its tensile integrity, insidious disc degeneration occurs. The individual may be without symptoms or may have multiple episodes of low back pain with a deep, vague, gnawing discomfort caused by proximal referred pain patterns. The patient may find that sitting is not as painful as standing, since the intradiscal pressures are reduced with the desiccation of the nucleus pulposus. Also, the facets may now begin to contribute to the individual's pain perception by becoming overloaded while the patient is standing in a lordotic posture, with the bisegmental innervation of the articular branch of the posterior rami providing the pertinent pain pathway (Fig. 1–26). In these circumstances, the x-rays may show only minimal disc space narrowing, at times with a vacuum phenomenon.

In either case, the intervertebral disc is no longer able to gracefully dissipate energy to the supporting muscles and ligaments and, particularly, to the posteriorly located facet joints and capsules. This eventually results in an x-ray appearance of degenerative joint disease of the spine, a disease that can result in the low back pain syndromes of lumbar spondylosis or degenerative arthritis, and in extreme cases, spinal stenosis with intermittent neurogenic claudication. Stiffness with immobilization, transient relief with ambulation, and insidious pain development with prolonged ambulation are the arthritic-type complaints that are encountered. The vague numbing sensation and lame weakness felt in the legs with ambulation and relieved by sitting represent the three-dimensional and postural encroachment on the spinal canal and foramina by hypertrophied facet joints, capsule laminae, and flavum that develop insidiously as disc incompetence evolves.

As with peripheral degenerative joint disease, the clinical, gross, and roentgenographic features may represent a primary disease state or a secondary phenomenon resulting from susceptible structural deficiencies that are either inherent or developmental. The appearance of degenerative joint disease may be more pronounced in those with familial tendencies for developing osteoarthritis, as has been demonstrated by the higher in-

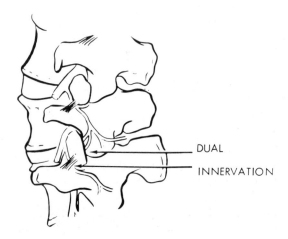

DUAL

INNERVATION

Figure 1–26. A lateral schematic of the spine showing the bisegmental innervation of the facet joints by the articular branch of von Luschka.

cidence of degenerative joint disease of the hip in patients with degenerative or type III spondylolisthesis of L4 or L5.[21] Those individuals who have a structural alteration of the spine caused by significant trauma, congenital defects, or poorly compensated scoliosis may have increased complaints because of developmental asymmetric loading of both disc and facet joints. The osteopenic spine, caused by osteoporosis, immobilization, osteomalacia, or some other form of metabolic bone disease, is susceptible to microfracture of the vertebral end-plate. This directly reduces the ability of the disc to dissipate energy by causing herniation of the nucleus into the substance of the weakened vertebral body or indirectly by reducing the mechanical ability of the disc by inhibiting the successful passage of nutrients through the compromised vertebral end-plate and its weakened subchondral scaffold. Undermining of the cartilage can also occur in the facet joints, thereby weakening motion segments anteriorly and posteriorly and making them more susceptible to degenerative change. The phenomenon can be exaggerated when a neuropathic component is superimposed on a structurally weakened component, as is the case of the classic Charcot's spine. Even simple articular trophism, which has been observed in cyclically loaded cadaver studies, may present a situation that completely changes the symmetric loading of the facets and that may therefore cause facet problems even when the intervertebral disc is still functioning adequately.[11]

AUTOIMMUNE CHANGES IN THE INTERVERTEBRAL DISC

The clinical syndromes of lumbar disc disease have been simplified by attributing biomechanical failure to biochemical alterations produced by inadequate nutrient delivery as the spine ages. The role of autoimmune disease in contributing to these syndromes and perhaps in accelerating the biochemical degeneration should be discussed.

The sequestered and avascular vitreous humor of the eye and the endocrine globulin of the thyroid gland are substances that, when released or exposed to the general circulation, can precipitate autoimmune phenomena known as sympathetic ophthalmia and Hashimoto's disease, respectively. These relatively avascular substances behave as antigens and trigger an inflammatory autoimmune response.[22] The relatively avascular intervertebral disc, however, has been implicated as an antigen trigger, when exposed to the vasculature by trauma, that promotes a more rapid degenerative process within the disc itself; this may also explain the inflammatory root syndrome or radiculitis seen in the absence of true disc herniation but also in conjunction with frank prolapse. It has been hypothesized (Fig. 1–27)[35] that, owing to the nutrient inadequacy of the intervertebral disc and the persistent demands or frank trauma at the annular end-plate interface made upon the susceptible biped spine, small fissures in the annulus can, with aging, expose some unknown antigen to the matrix maintenance cells of the annulus and the nucleus to the immune system. This sequence of events can cause the breakdown of lysosomal membranes,

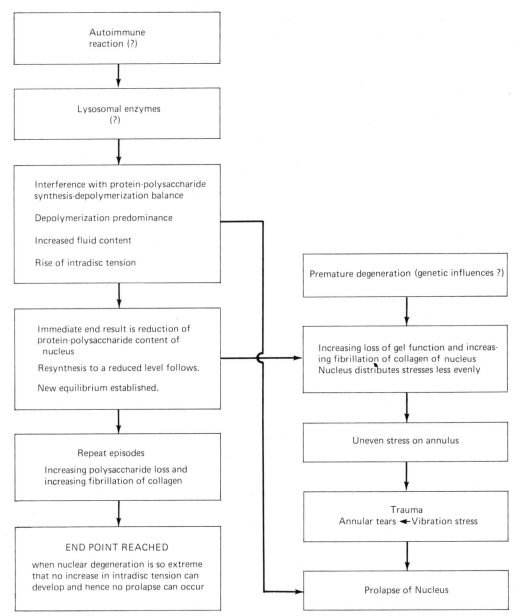

Figure 1–27. A schema by Naylor hypothesizing the autoimmune role in disc degeneration. (From Naylor, A.: Intervertebral disc. Spine, *1*:2, 1976.)

thereby releasing various enzymes that have been shown to degrade the glucosaminoglycan complexes of the intervertebral disc in vitro. It has also been demonstrated that the proteoglycans themselves have an antigen potential, particularly in the region of the attachment of the glucosamino-glycan to the protein core,[27] which is a clinically identifiable phenomenon in relapsing polychondritis.

Although various serum elevations of immunoglobulins M and G have been demonstrated in patients with surgically proven disc prolapses using the standard gel immunodiffusion plate, these immunoglobulins have not been demonstrated in disc tissue removed surgically.[32, 36] It is of further interest that the beta proteins mentioned earlier, which some observers feel represent debris from collagen breakdown, also have a roentgeno-graphic diffraction pattern similar to amyloid that may very well represent small chain alpha and kappa immunoglobulins.[36]

A cellular immune phenomenon, manifest through inhibition of leukocyte migration as well as lymphocyte transformation, has been demonstrated only on surgical cases in which the disc material has ruptured through the confines of the annulus and posterior ligament. Therefore, a sequestered disc can be thought of perhaps as "vascularized" by the general circulation and, in turn, may represent a significant antigen load.[15, 22]

There have been propositions that some as yet unknown protein complex representing debris from the matrix or fiber constituents of the intervertebral disc or an autoimmune antigen complex may be irritant to neural tissue, providing a more direct cause of the various lumbar disc syndromes.[35] Indeed, the branches of the posterior rami and the sinoverte-bral nerves, which are omnipresent and provide sensation to the annulus, epidural contents, muscles, ligaments, and facets, do provide an afferent pathway for pain perception (see Fig. 1–17). Unfortunately, because of this common pain pathway, annular rents, muscular strains, and ligament strains can all be manifest clinically as low back pain.

The susceptibility of the nerve roots to mechanical and chemical irritation has been explained in three different ways: (1) there is insuffi-cient epineurium around the roots, which ideally provides mechanical protection for peripheral nerves, (2) there are within the nerve root paral-lel and more susceptible orientations of the fasciculi compared to the peripheral nerve, and (3) the perineurium, which acts as a diffusion barrier against irritants in the peripheral nerve, is absent.[33] Therefore, on an immunologic basis, these three factors can explain the inflammatory susceptibility of the nerve root to an autoimmune phenomenon, with or without mechanical irritation, within the spinal canal or the neural fora-mina.

The favorable results[9, 12, 13, 24, 25, 45] reported in the treatment of sciati-ca and intermittent neurogenic claudication with oral steroids, intradiscal injections, and epidural steroids empirically support this concept in the pathophysiology of lumbar disc disease, but since these results have not been duplicated in double-blind studies,[6, 42] it is certainly possible that many factors can cause the various lumbar disc syndromes. It is also extremely difficult to explain the excellent results that can be obtained when an effective simple disc excision is performed, despite the nuclear material that remains within the confines of the intervertebral disc space.

Nevertheless, the chemical and mechanical changes that can be docu-mented in the spine grossly, histographically, roentgenographically, and biochemically appear to be phenomena that are universally tolerated or suffered by all to some degree as the spine ages. The clinical syndromes of lumbar disc disease, that is, the true pathophysiology of the lumbar disc, may be discussed with regard to the aging potential of the spine but can ultimately be explained only as the susceptibility of the anatomic pathways involved in and an individual's unique cortical perception of those painful stimuli. It is quite obvious that to discuss the pathophysiology of lumbar disc disease on purely anatomic, biochemical, and biomechanical terms without appreciating the complex cortical modulation of the patients themselves may lead only to diagnostic inadequacies and therapeutic disappointments.

REFERENCES

1. Adams, P., Eyre, D. R., and Muir, H.: Biochemical aspects of development and aging of human lumbar intervertebral discs. Rheum. Rehab., *16*:22, 1977.
2. Adams, P., and Muir, H.: Qualitative changes with age of proteoglycans of human lumbar disc. Ann. Rheum. Dis., *35*:289, 1976.
3. Arnold, C. C., et al.: Lumbar spinal stenosis and nerve root entrapment syndrome. Definition and classification. Clin. Orthop., *115*:4, 1976.
4. Barson, A. J. The vertebral level of termination of the spinal cord during normal and abnormal development. J. Anat., *106*:489, 1970.
5. Bernini, P., Wiesel, S., and Rothman, R.: Metrizamide myelography and the identification of anomalous lumbosacral nerve roots. J. Bone Joint Surg., *62A*:1203, 1980.
6. Bernini, P., Wiesel, S., and Rothman, R.: Unpublished data, 1979.
7. Brown, M., and Tsallas, T.: Studies on the permeability of the intervertebral disc during skeletal maturation. Spine, *4*:240, 1976.
8. Bushell, G. R., Ghosh, P., Taylor, F. F. K., and Akeson, W. H.: Proteoglycan chemistry of the intervertebral disks. Clin. Orthop., *129*:115, 1977.
9. Cappio, M.: Il Trattamento idrocortisonico per via epidurale sacrale delle lombosciatalgie. Reumatismo, *1*:60, 1957.
10. Coventry, M., Ghormley, R., and Kernohan, J. W.: The invertebral disc: its microscopic anatomy and pathology. Part I. J. Bone Joint Surg., *27*:105. Part II. J. Bone Joint Surg., *27*:233. Part III. J. Bone Joint Surg., *27*:460, 1945.
11. Cyron, D. M., and Hutton, W. C.: Articular tropism and stability of the lumbar spine. Spine, *5*:168, 1980.
12. D'Hooghe, R., Compere, A., Gribomont, B., and Vincent, A.: L'injection peridurale de corticosteroides dans le traitement du syndrome lombosciatalgique. Acta Orthopaedica Belgica, *42*:157, 1976.
13. Dilke, T. F. W., Burry, H. D., and Grahame, R.: Extradural corticosteroid injection in management of lumbar nerve root compression. Br. Med. J., *2*:635, 1973.
14. Dommisse, G. F.: The blood supply of the spinal cord. J. Bone Joint Surg., *56B*:225, 1974.
15. Elves, M., Bucknell, T., and Sullivan, M.: In vitro inhibition of leucocyte migration in patients with intervertebral disc lesions. Orthop. Clin. North Am., *6*:59, 1975.
16. Ericksen, M. F.: Aging in the lumbar spine. Am. J. Phys. Anthropol., *48*:241, 1974.
17. Farfan, H. F.: Mechanical Disorders of the Low Back. Philadelphia, Lee and Febiger, 1973.
18. Farfan, H. F., Osteria, V., and Lanry, C.: The mechanical etiology of spondylosis and spondylolisthesis. Clin. Orthop., *117*:40, 1976.
19. Feffer, H. L.: Regional use of steroids in the management of lumbar intervertebral disc disease. Orthop. Clin. North Am., *6*:249, 1975.
20. Feinstein, D., Langton, J.N. K., Jameson, R. M., and Schiller, F.: Experiments on pain referred from deep somatic tissues. J. Bone Joint Surg., *36A*:981, 1954.
21. Fitzgerald, J. A. W., and Newman, P. H.: Degenerative spondylolisthesis. J. Bone Joint Surg., *58B*:184, 1976.
22. Gertzbein, S. D., Tile, M., Gross, A., and Falk, R.: Autoimmunity in degenerative disc disease of the lumbar spine. Orthop. Clin. North Am., *6*:67, 1975.
23. Ghosh, R., Bushell, G. R., Taylor, T. F. K., and Akeson, W. H. Collagens, elastin and noncollagenous protein of the intervertebral disc. Clin. Orthop., *129*:124, 1977.
24. Goebert, H. W., Jr., Jallo, S. J., Gardner, W. J., and Wasmuth, C. E.: Painful radiculopathy. Anesth. Anal., *40*:130, 1961.
25. Green, L. N.: Dexamethasone in the management of symptoms due to herniated lumbar disc. J. Neurol. Neurosurg. Psychiatry, *38*:1211, 1975.

26. Hollinshead, W. H.: Anatomy for Surgeons, Vol. III. New York, Harper and Row, 1969.
27. Jayson, M., Herbert, C., and Darks, J.: Intervertebral disc: nuclear morphology and bursting pressures. Am. Rheum. Dis., *32*:308, 1973.
28. Keiser, A., and Sandson, J.: Immunology of cartilage proteoglycans. Fed. Proc., *32*:1474, 1972.
29. Kellgren, J. H.: The anatomical source of back pain. Rheum. Rehab., *16*:3, 1977.
30. Kulak, R. F., Belytschko, T. D., Schultz, A. D., and Galente, J. O.: Nonlinear behavior of the human intervertebral disc under axial load. J. Biomech., *9*:377, 1976.
31. Markoff, K. L., and Morris, J. M.: The structural components of the intervertebral disc. J. Bone Joint Surg., *56A*:675, 1974.
32. Marshall, L. L., Trethewie, E. R., and Curtain, C. C.: Chemical radiculitis. Clin. Orthop., *129*:61, 1977.
33. Murphy, M. D.: Nerve roots and spinal nerves in degenerative disk disease. Clin. Orthop., *129*:46, 1977.
34. Nachemson, A.: The load on lumbar disks in different positions of the body. Acta Orthop. Scand., *36*:426, 1965.
35. Naylor, A.: Intervertebral disc prolapse and degeneration. Spine, *1*:108, 1976.
36. Naylor, A., Happey, F., Turner, R. L., Stentall, R. D., West, D. C., and Richardson, C.: Enzymic and immunological activity in the intervertebral disc. Orthop. Clin. North Am., *6*:51, 1975.
37. O'Dell, C. W., Call, M., and Ignelzi, R.: Ascending lumbar venography in lumbar disc disease. J. Bone Joint Surg., *59A*:159, 1977.
38. Ogden, J.: Chondro-osseous development and teratology. Lecture X. Hilton Head Seminar. AAOS, 335–378, 1980.
39. Parke, W. W., Gammell, K., and Rothman, R.: Arterial vascularization of the cauda equina. J. Bone Joint Surg., *63A*:53, 1981.
40. Roth, M., Kirkoska, J., and Toman, I.: Morphogenesis of the spinal canal, normal and stenotic. Neuroradiology, *10*:277, 1976.
41. Schmorl, G., and Junghanns, H. The Human Spine in Health and Disease. New York and London, Grune and Stratton, 1971.
42. Snoek, W., Weber, H., and Jorgensen, B.: Double blind evaluation of extradural methylprednisolone for herniated lumbar discs. Acta Orthop. Scand., *48*:635, 1977.
43. Urban, J. P. G., Holm, S., Maroudas, A., and Nachemson, A.: Nutrition of the intervertebral disc. Clin. Orthop., *129*:101, 1977.
44. Vernon-Roberts, B., and Perie, C. J.: Degenerative changes in the intervertebral discs of the lumbar spine and their sequelae. Rheum. Rehab., *16*:13, 1977.
45. Warr, A. C., Wilkinson, J. A., Burn, J. M. B., and Langdon, L.: Chronic lumbosciatica syndrome treated by epidural injection and manipulation. Practitioner, *209*:53, 1972.
46. Wiltse, L. L., Neuman, P. H., and Macnal, I.: Classification of spondylolysis and spondylolisthesis. Clin. Orthop., *117*:23, 1976.

Chapter 2

DIAGNOSTIC STUDIES IN EVALUATING DISEASE AND AGING IN THE LUMBAR SPINE

ROUTINE RADIOGRAPHY

Radiographic examination of the lumbar spine is considered an integral part of the examination of the patient with signs and symptoms of lumbar spine pathology. It should be emphasized, however, that the radiographic examination is only one facet of the total picture and that the treating physician should not allow his judgment to be superseded by the x-ray. Degenerative changes involving the facet joints or the vertebral body/intervertebral disc complex cannot definitely be seen as either causative of low back pain syndrome[34, 51] or predictive as to the development of low lumbar complaints.[29] In cases of degenerative spondylolisthesis, which is an advanced manifestation of both disc degeneration and degenerative subluxation of the facet joints, many patients are essentially symptom-free.[15] Conversely, in young patients, a marked disc prolapse with incapacitating pain may be present in the face of a completely normal x-ray.

The radiograph must be of excellent quality and taken with great attention to detail. It should routinely include anteroposterior, lateral, and oblique views (see Fig. 1–13). Special views will be necessary if visualization of the sacroiliac joints is indicated (Table 2–1).

Thinning or loss of height of the disc space is frequently seen in disc degeneration. DePalma and Rothman found in cases of operatively proven disc degeneration at L5 that there was radiographic evidence of disc space narrowing in 41 per cent of cases. In cases of disc degeneration at L4, radiographic evidence of disc space narrowing occurs in 19 per cent of cases.[8] It should be emphasized that thinning of the disc space, although an indication of disc degeneration, may be noted at a level other than that producing the presenting symptoms and may not be present at all. It should also be recalled that narrowing of the disc space is not unique to disc degeneration but may also occur in metabolic and infectious diseases of vertebral motion segments. Narrowing is also frequently seen below a transitional lumbosacral vertebra and represents a vestigial intervertebral disc that is rarely, if ever, symptomatic (Fig. 2–1).[54]

There is a greater incidence of degenerative changes in the lumbar

TABLE 2–1. Roentgenographic Differential Diagnosis of the Hyperostotic Spine

Site	Ankylosing Hyperostosis of the Spine	Ankylosing Spondylitis	Degenerative Osteoarthritis
Vertebral Body and Intervertebral Disc	A continual "flowing" and variably thickened outgrowth of bone on the anterolateral aspect of all the vertebral bodies. There is a predilection for the dorsal lumbar region, particularly on the right side, with good preservation of disc space height.	Relatively thin syndesmophytes anteriorly with squaring of the vertebral bodies while preserving good disc space height.	Sclerosis of superior and inferior surfaces of the vertebral body with osteophytic lipping associated with moderate to severe decrease in disc space height and with occasional vacuum phenomenon.
Zygapophyseal Joints	Normal or mild sclerosis with occasional osteophytes.	Erosions, sclerosis, and bony ankylosis.	Normal or sclerotic with occasional hypertrophic changes.
Sacroiliac Joints	Preserved.	Erosions with bony ankylosis.	Usually preserved.

motion segments with increasing age,[29, 33, 51] which is exemplified by decreased vertebral height and increased vertebral width,[11, 12] sclerosis of the subchondral bone, and formation of peripheral osteophytes with disc degeneration (Fig. 2–2).[25] Bone spurs are not pathognomonic of disc degeneration but must be differentiated from other conditions such as Reiter's syndrome, ankylosing spondylitis,[10] and ankylosing hyperostosis of the spine.[6] Osteophytes are usually more prominent anterolaterally than posterolaterally, and their presentation is most likely a result of the nature of the annulus and ligamentous attachments to the bodies of the vertebrae above and below the degenerative disc space.[51] McNab has described a unique horizontal osteophyte found 2 to 3 millimeters from the disc space. which he terms the "traction spur." This is thought to arise from stress at the site of the ligamentous insertion during the hypermobile phase of disc degeneration (Figs. 2–3 and 2–4).[32]

The sclerosis seen adjacent to the end-plate of the vertebra may be a thin, diffuse zone, or it may be localized anteriorly or posteriorly. Occasionally, a considerable portion of the vertebra will be involved, which can simulate a neoplastic or infectious process (Fig. 2–5).

Disc herniations may occur directly into the body of the vertebrae (Schmorl's nodes) (see Fig. 1–11) and are most commonly seen in the upper lumbar and lower thoracic areas, with frequency varying as a function of the investigative techniques used.[41] They occur most often in the central and posterocentral portion of the body, surrounded by sclerotic bone. In all likelihood, the herniation follows the notochordal or vascular residual channels or both through the cartilaginous vertebral end-plate. There may also be a limbus vertebra, which is described as an anterosuperior herniation that results in a triangular segment of vertebra becoming separated from the parent bone by the displaced nucleus pulposus (Fig. 2–6).[21, 43] A relative weakness at the interface of the vertebral

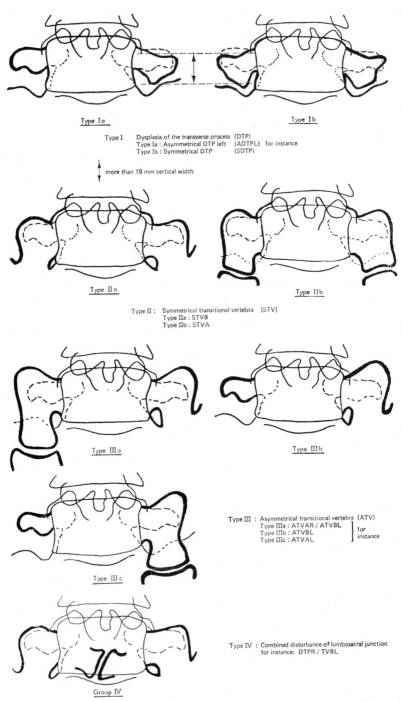

Type Ia

Type Ib

Type I Dysplasia of the transverse process (DTP)
Type Ia : Asymmetrical DTP left (ADTPL) for instance
Type Ib : Symmetrical DTP (SDTP)

more than 19 mm vertical width

Type IIa

Type IIb

Type II : Symmetrical transitional vertebra (STV)
Type IIa : STVB
Type IIb : STVA

Type IIIa

Type IIIb

Type III : Asymmetrical transitional vertebra (ATV)
Type IIIa : ATVAR / ATVBL
Type IIIb : ATVBL for instance
Type IIIc : ATVAL

Type IIIc

Group IV

Type IV : Combined disturbance of lumbosacral junction
for instance: DTPR / TVBL

Figure 2–1. Classification of lumbosacral transitional vertebra. (From Timmi, P. G., Wieser, C., and Zinn, W.: The transitional vertebra of the lumbosacral spine: Its radiological classification, incidence, prevalence, and clinical significance. Rheumatol. Rehabil. *16*:180, 1977.)

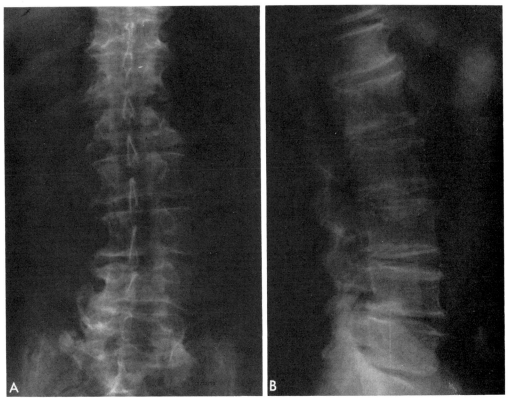

Figure 2–2. Radiographs of the lumbar spine illustrate advanced multilevel disc degeneration with loss of height of the disc space, marked osteophyte formation, and sclerosis of the end plates. Foraminal encroachment is present. (From Rothman, R. H., and Simeone, F. A.: The Spine, 2nd ed. Philadelphia, W. B. Saunders Co., 1982.)

body and cartilaginous end-plate may predispose an individual to this type of herniation. Although there is no correlation between this type of pathology and posterior herniations causing spinal nerve encroachment, an association with disc disease has been suggested.[27]

The differential diagnosis should also include pathologic states such as trauma, infection, congenital defects, or metabolic disease, which may weaken the cartilaginous end-plate or the vertebral body itself and subsequently allow for an intravertebral herniation.[41]

During the course of disc degeneration, derangements in the alignment of vertebrae may occur as well as alterations in their normal motion. A particular motion unit, that is, the disc and its two adjacent vertebrae, will often go through a hypermobile phase (Fig. 2–7) early in the course of disc degeneration and at a later stage achieve a hypomobile phase with focal suppression of motion. There is a wide variation in this tendency, but the end-point roentgenographic appearance is referred to as a type III or degenerative spondylolisthesis (Fig. 2–8). The tendency toward anterior migration (pseudospondylolisthesis) or posterior migration (pseudoretrospondylolisthesis) of one vertebral body over the subjacent vertebra is a function of the total force vector acting differently on separate motion units throughout the lumbar space. The degree and direction of the

Text continued on page 42

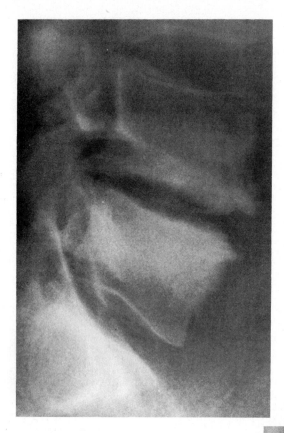

Figure 2-3. Traction osteophyte at the L4–5 level associated with disc degeneration. Note sclerosis at the adjacent vertebral bodies and narrowing of the disc space. (From Rothman, R. H., and Simeone, F. A.: The Spine, 2nd ed. Philadelphia, W. B. Saunders Co., 1982.)

Figure 2-4. Traction osteophyte at the L3–4 level. Note that the osteophyte is horizontally oriented and 2 mm. away from the disc space. Note the marked narrowing of the disc space and the vacuum phenomenon at L3–4. (From Rothman, R. H. and Simeone, F. A.: The Spine, 2nd ed. Philadelphia, W. B. Saunders Co., 1982.)

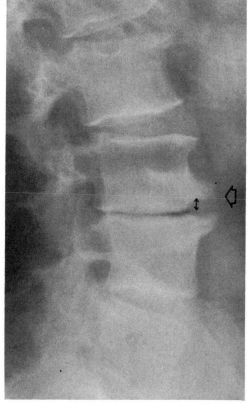

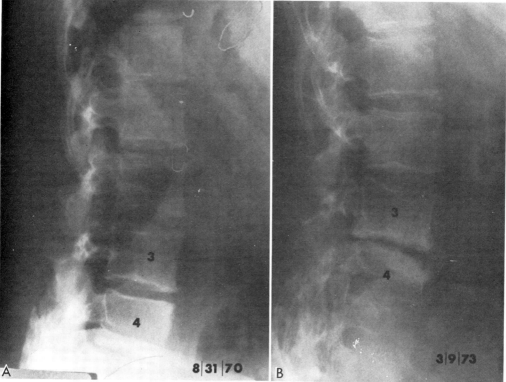

Figure 2–5. Radiographs illustrate the development of disc degeneration at the L3-L4 disc space over a period of three years. Note the loss of height of the disc space, osteophyte formation, and sclerosis of the end plates. In this instance the radiographic appearance was suggestive of infection, and biopsy was performed but revealed only evidence of chronic disc degeneration. At times the sclerosis can be so marked as to simulate a neoplasm of the vertebral body. (From Rothman, R. H., and Simeone, F. A.: The Spine, 2nd ed. Philadelphia, W. B. Saunders Co., 1982.)

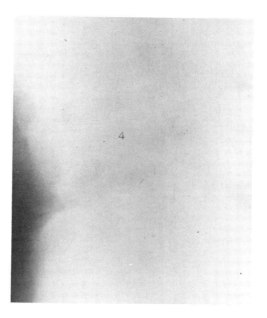

Figure 2–6. A limbus vertebra. The diastasis between L4 and the supra-anterior corner of that vertebra is realized by an interposing amount of nucleus pulposus.

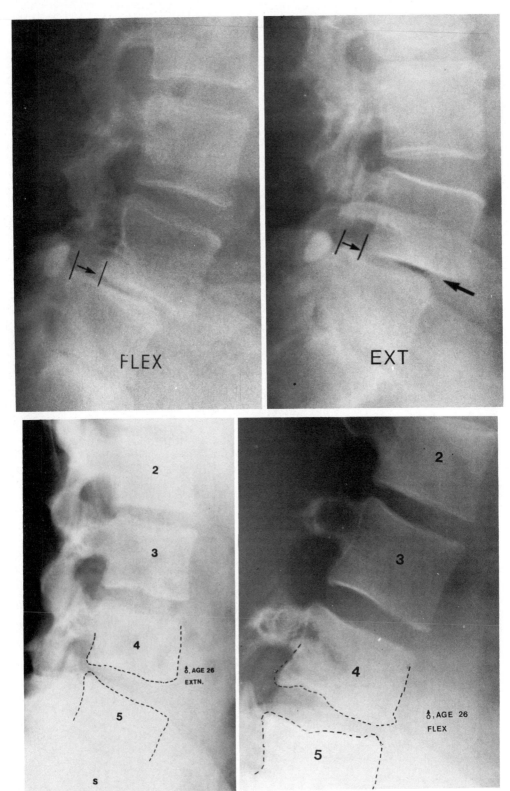

Figure 2–7. Manifestations of sagittal as well as angular instability in the hypermobile phase of disc degeneration and facet subluxation. (From Rothman. R. H., and Simeone, F. A.: The Spine, 2nd ed. Philadelphia, W. B. Saunders Co., 1982.)

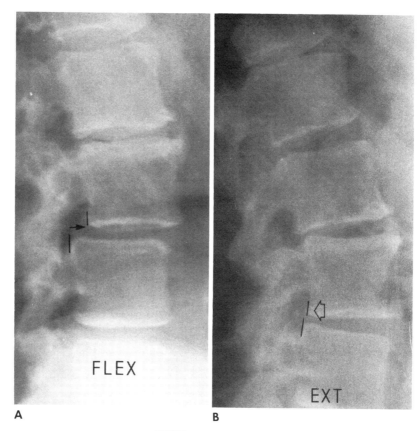

A

B

FLEX

EXT

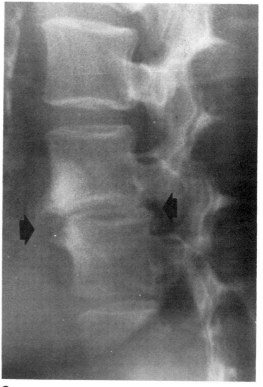

C

Figure 2–8. Radiographs illustrate segmental instability due to disc degeneration on flexion and extension views. *A,* Note that in flexion there is a 3.5-mm. anterior migration of the cranial vertebra. *B,* In extension there is almost complete realignment of the vertebral body. This was productive of both back pain and sciatica. *C,* Radiograph illustrates marked disc degeneration at the L3–4 level. There is associated loss of height of the disc space, sclerosis of the adjacent vertebral body, osteophyte formation, and a 2-mm. retrospondylolisthesis. (From Rothman, R. H., and Simeone, F. A.: The Spine, 2nd ed. Philadelphia, W. B. Saunders Co., 1982.)

Lumbar (L1 to L5) Spine

Element	Point Value
Cauda equina damage	3
Relative flexion sagittal plane translation 8%	
or extension sagittal plane translation 9%	2
Relative flexion sagittal plane rotation 9°	2
Anterior elements destroyed	2
Posterior elements destroyed	2
Dangerous loading anticipated	1
Total of 5 or more = clinically unstable	

Lumbosacral (L5 to S1) Spine

Element	Point Value
Cauda equina damage	3
Relative flexion sagittal plane translation 6%	
or extension sagittal plane translation 9%	2
Relative flexion sagittal plane rotation 1%	2
Anterior elements destroyed	2
Posterior elements destroyed	2
Dangerous loading anticipated	1
Total of 5 or more = clinically unstable	

Figure 2–9. Checklists for the diagnosis of clinical instability in the lumbar spine and at the lumbosacral junction. Cauda equina damage is worth three points, including two points for destruction of all posterior or anterior elements, and one point in cases where dangerous loads are expected. Instability is diagnosed by the presence of five or more points, according to the checklists. (From Posner, I., White, A. A., Edwards, W. T., and Hayes, W. C.: Spinal Stability Criteria, Lumbar Spine. Presented before the Eastern Orthopaedic Association, 1980.)

spondylolisthesis depend on the amount of degenerative "disease" that has occurred, the inherent soft tissue stability that is present, and the segment of the lordotic lumbar spine that is involved. Guidelines have been provided by Posner and White[38] and others to quantify instability, but these guidelines have not yet been clinically correlated with all lumbar symptoms (Fig. 2–9).

Allbrook,[2] Farfan et al.,[14] and Fitzgerald and Newman[15] emphasize the importance of the iliotransverse ligament (which runs from the transverse process of L5 to the iliac crest) in inhibiting spondylolisthesis by acting as a guidewire in the lower vertebral segments. Furthermore, they have demonstrated that a deep-seated lumbar spine within the confines of the iliac wings will tend to put increased stress on the L4–L5 motion segment and contribute to the greater incidence of degenerative spondylolisthesis generally found at that level (see Fig. 2–7).

The hallmark of this phenomenon, however, is slow, insidious degeneration of the disc and subluxation of the facet joints, referred to as the "articular bolt" by Taillard.[49] These changes in alignment may produce significant symptoms of radiculopathy or intermittent neurogenic claudication, particularly in a congenitally narrow spinal canal. If this occurs at L3–L4 or L4–L5, the clinician will not uncommonly see a complete myelographic block resulting from the phenomenon, even though the spondylolisthesis will minimally range from a few millimeters to 1 to 1.5

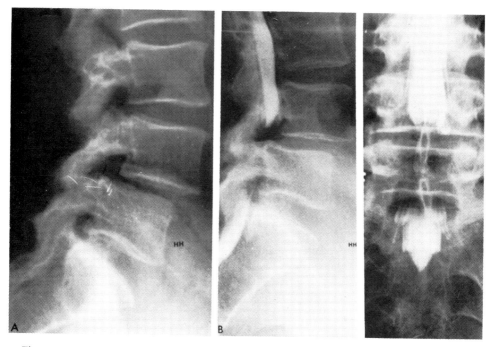

Figure 2–10. Metrizamide myelogram shows stenotic block at the L4–5 level due to degenerative spondylolisthesis and spinal stenosis at the L4–5 level. *A*, Note the 4-mm. anterior migration of L4 on L5 owing to the degenerative spondylolisthesis. *B*, Note the extensive block on the metrizamide myelogram owing to this spinal stenosis. (From Rothman, R. H., and Simeone, F. A.: The Spine, 2nd ed. Philadelphia, W. B. Saunders Co., 1982.)

cm. or up to 33 per cent with an average slip of 17 per cent (Fig. 2–10).[15, 49]

Encroachment of the intervertebral foramina occurs, but it should be realized that the spatial relationships are such that more leeway is present for the nerve root or the spinal nerve in the lumbar foramina than in the cervical area. The dynamic compromise of the foramina with lordosis, which is exaggerated in extension, in conjunction with posterior osteophytes, hypertrophy or redundancy of capsular ligaments, subluxation of the facets, and narrowing of the disc space with approximation of the pedicle will jointly affect the exiting spinal nerves and the theca (Fig. 2–11). The spinal nerve rests in the uppermost portion of the foramina, usually well above the disc space, but the tip of the superior facet may impinge on the spinal nerve as it subluxes in a cranial direction. In the presence of concomitant olisthesis, the foraminal compromise is increased.

Calcification of the nucleus does not occur often in lumbar disc degeneration, but it may be noted in the annulus fibrosus. Ratheke,[40] in a postmortem study of human spines, found this type of calcification present in 71 per cent of the spines examined. Magnussen[33] first called attention to the so-called "vacuum phenomenon" as a sign of disc degeneration (see Fig. 2–4). The vacuum phenomenon, which is accentuated in extension

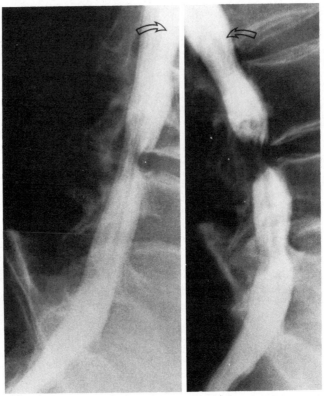

Figure 2–11. Metrizamide myelogram with flexion-extension lateral views reveals a partial block in flexion and a complete block in extension. Patient became markedly paretic in extension. This illustrates classic spinal stenosis secondary to disc degeneration. (From Rothman, R. H., and Simeone, F. A.: The Spine, 2nd ed. Philadelphia, W. B. Saunders Co., 1982.)

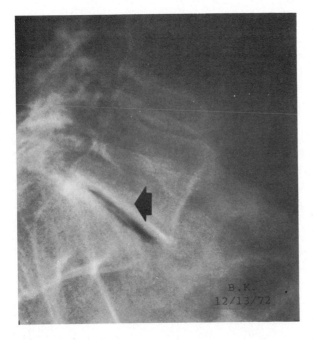

Figure 2–12. Radiograph illustrates the vacuum phenomenon at the L5–S1 disc space due to release of dissolved gas during extension stress on the spine. (From Rothman, R. H., and Simeone, F. A.: The Spine, 2nd ed. Philadelphia, W. B. Saunders Co., 1982.)

and diminished or eliminated in flexion of the spine, permits the free diffusion of primarily nitrogen from the extracellular fluid into the nuclear recesses of the degenerative disc (Fig. 2–12).[16]

As previously noted, the stigmata of disc degeneration, with and without transitional vertebrae, are seen in a very large percentage of the population, many of whom have no symptoms referable to their lumbar spine. For this reason, the stigmata should be considered significant only when symptoms are present, and they should be carefully correlated with the individual's history and physical examination.

MYELOGRAM

General Concepts

A carefully performed myelogram is an invaluable aid in the surgical treatment of various diseases of the lumbar spine, and the authors feel that this study should be performed in most instances before surgical intervention is undertaken. The rationale for performing myelography is based on the following advantages.

Myelography may demonstrate tumors of the spinal cord that can clinically mimic symptomatic disc disease. Several striking examples have been seen in which the history and neurologic findings were characteristic of a herniated lumbar disc at the L4 or L5 level, and yet, to the surprise of the treating surgeon, a myelogram revealed a tumor of the lower thoracic or upper lumbar spine. Although the demonstration of a disc herniation occurring simultaneously with an intradural or intramedullary tumor is rare, the possibility remains. The authors also feel that, in addition to myelography, cerebrospinal fluid (CSF) protein analysis should be performed at the time of lumbar puncture. The wary surgeon may be steered away from inappropriate surgery and unsatisfactory results when an abnormal myelogram that may be consistent with an intradural or epidural defect is viewed in combination with a markedly elevated CSF protein level.

A second advantage of routine myelography is that a more exact localization of disc herniation and spinal nerve compromise can be determined. Edgar and Park[13] proposed a dual coordinate approach to diagnosing symptomatic lumbar disc disease. Although they could accurately predict the horizontal location (either central, posterolateral, or lateral) of a disc herniation in 80 per cent of cases in this prospective study with a straight leg raising test, the vertical coordinate or level was identified without the use of myelography only 50 per cent of the time. Hakelius and Hindmarsh[24] found a comparable 46 per cent accuracy rate as to the involved level prediction on the basis of neurologic findings alone. Indeed, a variation in the nerve root configuration (i.e., nerve root anomalies) (Fig. 2–13) and the location of the extrusion can lead to erroneous decisions if neurologic deficit alone is considered. An axillary or central protrusion at the L4 level may cause the S1 spinal nerve syndrome that is usually characteristic of an L5 protrusion. Conversely, a very lateral L4 herniation

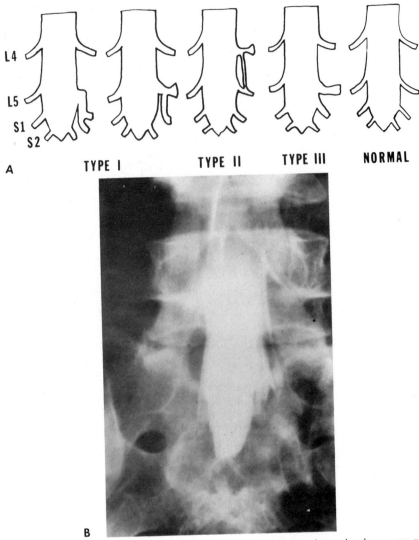

Figure 2–13. *A,* Diagram of the three types of anomalous lower lumbar nerve roots, with a normal root for comparison (modified from a figure by Cannon et al.). (From Bernini, P. M., Wiesel, S. W., and Rothman, R. H.: Metrizamide myelography and the identification of anomalous lumbosacral nerve roots. J. Bone Joint Surg., *62A*:1203, 1980.) *B,* Anomalous nerve root, type 1. Note the conjoined nerve root exiting beneath the first sacral pedicle in a patient who had both L5 and S1 symptoms and signs.

or a central herniation with cranial migration of the fragment may cause an L4 spinal nerve syndrome rather than the expected L5 syndrome. Double disc herniations (that is, at more than one level) can result in a confusing neurologic picture that may not be clarified and appropriately treated without myelographic definition (Fig. 2–14).

A literature review[19] revealed an overall myelographic accuracy rate of 85 per cent. The shortcomings of this study were more often in sensitivity (false negative) than in specificity (false positive). Improved accuracy of myelography is seen with the newer water-soluble dyes (see following

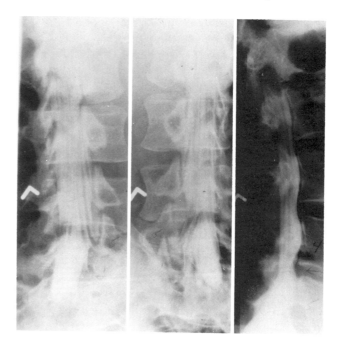

Figure 2–14. A double disc herniation correlated with both L5 and S1 radicular complaints.

section). Even the more viscous oil-based dye should obviate the need for multiple level explorations if used in the proper clinical setting.

It should be emphasized that the definition afforded by myelography can be completely realized only by proper technique and a complete series of exposures that includes anteroposterior and oblique as well as standing and prone laterals. Flexion-extension films may also increase the yield, particularly when symptoms are dynamically exaggerated.

WATER-SOLUBLE VERSUS OIL LUMBAR MYELOGRAPHY

Although oil myelography has traditionally been used in this country, Food and Drug Administration (FDA) approval of the water-soluble agent metrizamide in 1978 has made this contrast material the preferred agent for lumbar spine studies. Radiopaque water-soluble contrast media have been used extensively in arteriography and intravenous pyelography and in a variety of radiologic tests in order to visualize internal organs. When injected into the subarachnoid space, these substances are absorbed in a few hours.[22] In light of the well-established relationship between symptomatic arachnoiditis and oil-based myelography, particularly when associated with surgical intervention,[48] efforts were made to develop less toxic contrast media. A variety of water-soluble media were used during the 1940s and 1950s, but all were too toxic for investigative use in humans. Contact with the spinal cord or nerve roots induced permanent damage, and extreme pain was associated with their use.

Metrizamide (Amipaque), a water-soluble triionate contrast medium, was developed in Norway to overcome the shortcomings of the earlier developed water-soluble dyes. Unlike other water-soluble dyes, metrizamide is nonionic and does not dissociate and therefore provides lower osmolality in solution. Although it is slightly hyperbaric, its isotonicity (when used with a suggested iodine concentration of 170 mg. per ml.) has been suggested as the reason for its causing fewer adverse effects and, in particular, less arachnoiditis.[23, 42] To date, there have been no radiographically proven cases of arachnoiditis from the use of metrizamide.

Our experience regarding patient tolerance of the dye has been excellent; although headaches, nausea, and vomiting are not infrequent, they are transient side-effects reported with similar incidence elsewhere.[3, 4] Most recently, however, these adverse effects have been diminished when special attention is given to the hydration of the patient orally and intravenously prior to the study.

In addition to the acceptable level of short- and long-term adverse signs and symptoms associated with metrizamide, this contrast material has provided a more facile technique of myelography and better resolution of the theca and the spinal nerves than has been appreciated with oil contrast media. The preoperation identification of anomalous nerve roots is now possible owing to the low viscosity of metrizamide. The subarachnoid extension of the nerve root sleeves can be easily traced within the foramen rather than having to stop at the shoulder of the sleeve, as was so frequently encountered with oil-based myelography.[5]

Because metrizamide is absorbed through the lumbar theca and primarily through the parasagittal arachnoid villae over the brain, removal of the dye is not required; therefore, the most time-consuming and uncomfortable part of the oil myelographic procedure is avoided.

The fully miscible metrizamide provides an excellent delineation of the subarachnoid extension of each spinal nerve into the neural foramina as well as of the entire cauda equina stemming from the easily identifiable conus. Even subtle changes in the dimension or shape of a spinal nerve may be of significance if they fit the clinical presentation. Dynamic studies and supine filming are obviously easier, since the spinal needle can be removed after dye injection (because dye removal is obviated with this contrast medium).

Because of its slow absorption (approximately 1 ml. per year), the authors may still use oil-soluble contrast media with a steroid preparation with individuals who have definitely confirmed iodine allergies. However, use of the fourth generation computerized axial tomogram has reduced the need for oil-soluble contrast even more. In cases in which prolonged lower thoracic exposures are required or acute cauda equina syndrome develops, however, oil contrast is still preferred.

ABNORMAL PATTERNS OF MYELOGRAPHY

Various patterns of myelographic abnormalities are noted, depending on the size and location of the protrusion as well as the contrast material that is used. Soft disc herniations will present a much different pattern

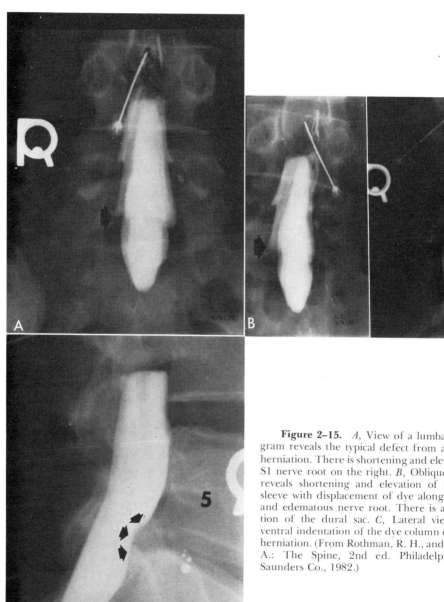

Figure 2–15. *A,* View of a lumbar oil myelogram reveals the typical defect from a lateral disc herniation. There is shortening and elevation of the S1 nerve root on the right. *B,* Oblique view again reveals shortening and elevation of the S1 root sleeve with displacement of dye along the swollen and edematous nerve root. There is also indentation of the dural sac. *C,* Lateral view reveals a ventral indentation of the dye column due to a disc herniation. (From Rothman, R. H., and Simeone, F. A.: The Spine, 2nd ed. Philadelphia, W. B. Saunders Co., 1982.)

than the defects that are noted with chronic disc degeneration and osteophyte formation (spinal stenosis).

Posterolateral Disc Herniations

The defects that are most often noted with posterolateral disc herniations are incomplete filling or elevation of the spinal nerve sleeve, lateral indentation of the dural sac, and double density of the sac noted in the lateral view. A large lateral herniation may also produce a complete myelographic block at the level of the disc space. Elevation of the nerve sleeve may be the only abnormality noted in the lateral disc protrusion, but it is the least reliable of the findings. This is particularly true in oil myelography, since the viscoid material may occasionally fail to completely fill the normal nerve sleeve. Owing to improved radicular definition with metrizamide, subtle changes in the contour or location of the spinal nerve are more meaningful, particularly if there is asymmetric proximal swelling of the nerve within the central dye column. Indentation of the dural sac seen in the anteroposterior or oblique view and the double density seen in the lateral view with either contrast medium are more convincing findings (Figs. 2–15 to 2–18).

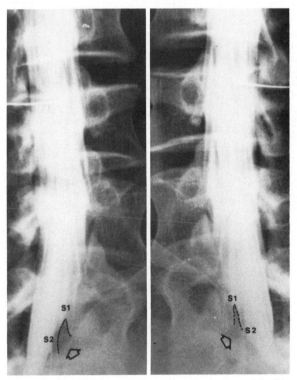

Figure 2–16. Metrizamide myelogram illustrating asymmetry of the S1 spinal nerve due to axillary herniation at L5–S1 on the left. (From Rothman, R. H., and Simeone, F. A.: The Spine, 2nd ed. Philadelphia, W. B. Saunders Co., 1982.)

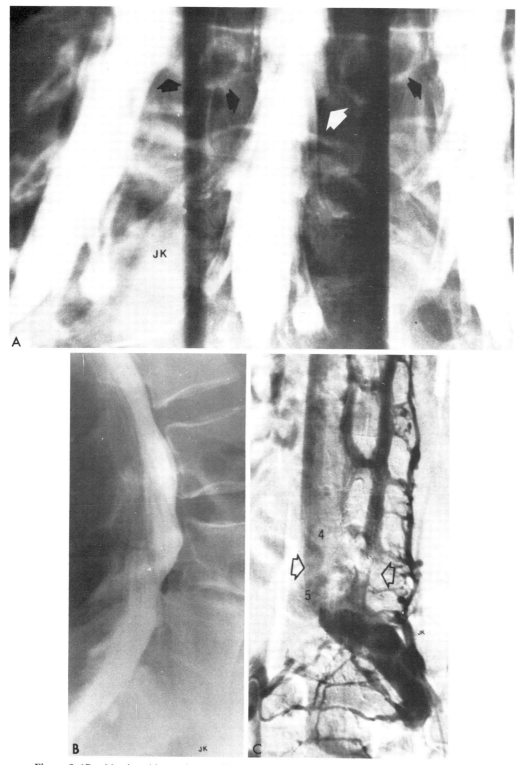

Figure 2–17. Metrizamide myelogram illustrating a herniated disc at the L4–5 level on the right. *A*, Note obliteration of the nerve root sleeve and indentation of the dural sac. *B*, Lateral view illustrates ventral indentation of the dural sac. *C*, Epidural venogram reveals occlusion of the anterior internal vertebral vein and radicular vein at the L4–5 level on the right. (From Rothman, R. H., and Simeone, F. A.: The Spine, 2nd ed. Philadelphia, W. B. Saunders Co., 1982.)

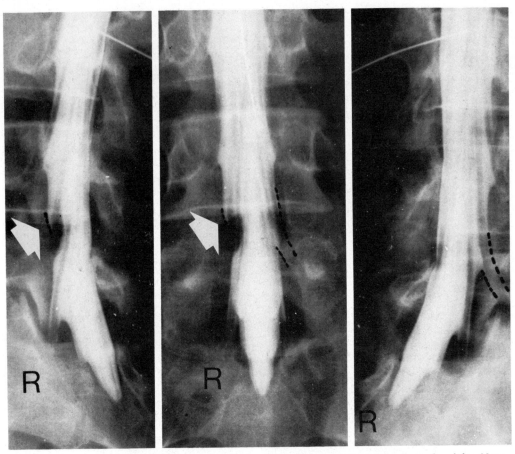

Figure 2–18. Metrizamide myelogram illustrating a herniated disc at L4–5 on the right. Note amputation of the nerve root sleeve and indentation of the dural sac. (From Rothman, R. H., and Simeone, F. A.: The Spine, 2nd ed. Philadelphia, W B. Saunders Co., 1982.)

Central Herniations

Large central disc herniations will often produce a characteristic complete myelographic block. The block will occur at the level of the disc space and, in the anteroposterior view, will show an irregular sawtooth or paintbrush appearance. The lateral view will reveal the anterior portion of the dural sac being compressed and elevated owing to ventral pressure from the disc herniation. A stenotic effect is commonly noticed with smaller central discs as the origins of the nerve sleeves are forced laterally, preventing the dye from filling this area. More often than not, however, such "wasp-waisting" defects are more compatible with roentgenographic spinal stenosis, with or without contributing disc herniation (Figs. 2–19, 2–20).

Free Fragments

Free fragments of disc material may migrate in either a caudal or a cranial direction and will be seen as well-circumscribed masses of varying diameters at a distance from the disc space (Figs. 2–21, 2–22).

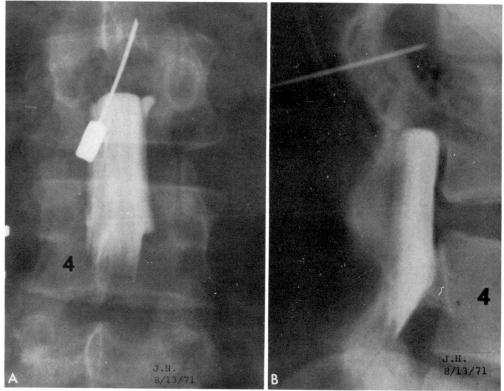

Figure 2–19. *A*, This oil myelogram illustrates a large central disc herniation. The antero-posterior view reveals a complete block at the L4–5 level, with an irregular sawtooth or paintbrush appearance characteristic of the block defect produced by disc herniation. *B*, Lateral view of the same patient reveals characteristic block pattern due to disc herniation with ventral pressure on the dye column producing a complete block at the level of the large central disc herniation. (From Rothman, R. H., and Simeone, F. A.: The Spine, 2nd ed. Philadelphia, W. B. Saunders Co., 1982.)

Spinal Stenosis: Chronic Disc Degeneration

Chronic disc degeneration will frequently be associated with spinal stenosis and will often produce myelographic defects caused by diffuse posterior bulging of the annulus, hypertrophy and redundancy of capsular and ligamentous tissue, and osteophyte formation. In the anteroposterior views, a symmetric waisting of the dye column will be noted, resulting from obliteration of the lateral recess. In the lateral views, the indentation of the dye column at the level of the disc space will be seen. If no osteophytes are present, the dye indentation will usually be 2 to 3 mm. in height; if osteophytes are present, they are easily seen and coincide with the defect in the dye column (Figs. 2–23 to 2–30).

Artifacts

Many artifacts present in myelography can create defects that are not truly representative of disc degeneration. The defect created by the spinal

Text continued on page 61

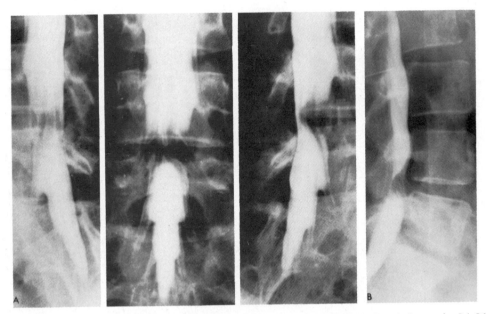

Figure 2–20.   This metrizamide myelogram illustrates a large central disc herniation at the L4–L5 level. *A,* Anteroposterior and oblique views reveal this prominent defect more marked on the right. *B,* This lateral view illustrates a "double density" prominent ventral indentation of the dye column. (From Rothman, R. H., and Simeone, F. A.: The Spine, 2nd ed. Philadelphia, W. B. Saunders Co., 1982.)

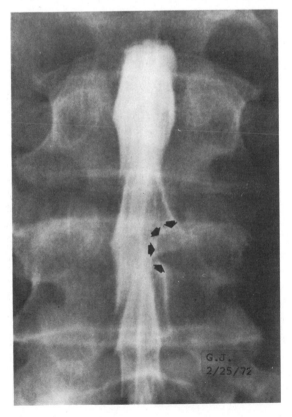

Figure 2–21.   Free fragments of disc material produce a myelographic defect characterized by smooth, well-circum-scribed indentations in the dye column. They may be at the level of the disc space or migrate at a distance. They may be difficult to differentiate from neurofibro-mata. Oil was the contrast medium in this illustration. (From Rothman, R. H., and Simeone, F. A.: The Spine, 2nd ed. Phila-delphia, W. B. Saunders Co., 1982.)

Figure 2–22. Metrizamide myelogram illustrates a disc herniation with cephalic migration of a free fragment anterior to the mid-portion of the body of L3 on the left. Note swelling of the L3 root and absence of the L4 root. The patient had marked quadriceps atrophy and absence of patellar reflex. (From Rothman, R. H., and Simeone, F. A.: The Spine, 2nd ed. Philadelphia, W. B. Saunders Co., 1982.)

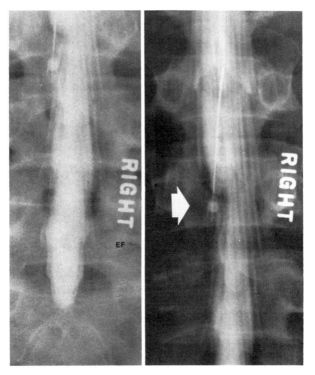

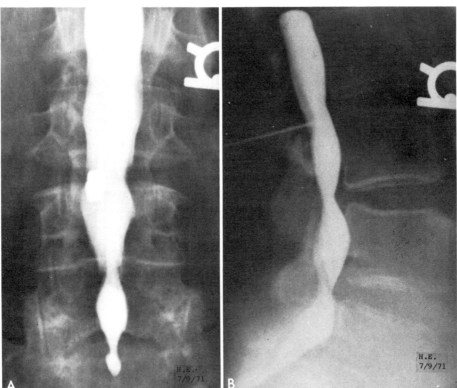

Figure 2–23. Oil myelograms show the characteristic appearance of chronic disc degeneration and spinal stenosis with diffuse posterior bulging of the annulus and osteophyte formation. There is symmetrical waisting of the dye column in the A-P view. The lateral view will show indentation of the dye column by the annulus anteriorly and the buckled ligamentum flavum and facet joints posteriorly. (From Rothman, R. H., and Simeone, F. A.: The Spine, 2nd ed. Philadelphia, W. B. Saunders Co., 1982.)

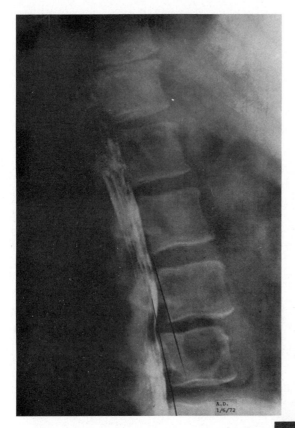

Figure 2–24. Flexion view of the lumbar spine reveals marked anterior migration of L3 on L4 secondary to disc degeneration. This is termed degenerative spondylolisthesis or pseudospondylolisthesis. (From Rothman, R. H., and Simeone, F A.: The Spine, 2nd ed. Philadelphia, W. B. Saunders Co., 1982.)

Figure 2–25. Myelogram reveals a complete block at the level of L3–L4 secondary to the pseudospondylolisthesis seen in Figure 2–24. (From Rothman, R. H., and Simeone, F. A.: The Spine, 2nd ed. Philadelphia, W. B. Saunders Co., 1982.)

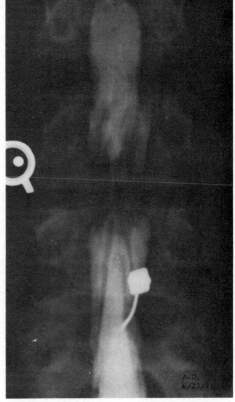

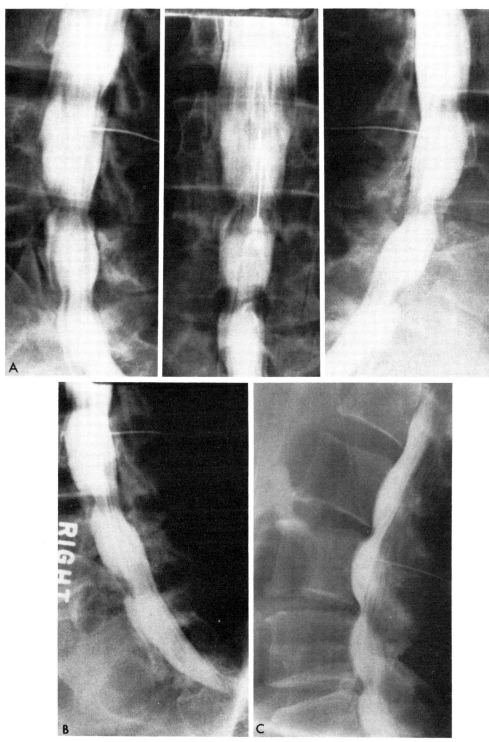

Figure 2–26. Metrizamide myelogram reveals this multiple-level spinal stenosis secondary to disc degeneration. *A* and *B*, The anteroposterior and oblique views reveal the multiple waisting defects typical of spinal stenosis. *C*, Lateral view illustrates multiple ventral defects due to diffuse bulging at the annulus. (From Rothman, R. H., and Simeone, F. A.: The Spine, 2nd ed. Philadelphia, W. B. Saunders Co., 1982.)

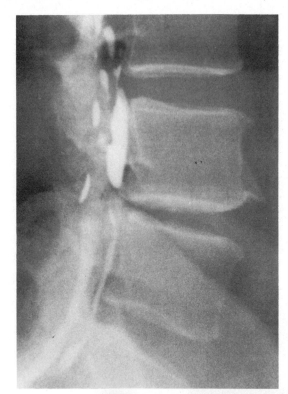

Figure 2–27. This oil myelogram reveals a complete block at the L4–5 level on the lateral view due to spinal stenosis. Note the traction osteophyte anteriorly associated with narrowing of the disc space and enlargement of the facet joints. The block is at the level of the disc space. (From Rothman, R. H., and Simeone, F. A.: The Spine, 2nd ed. Philadelphia, W. B. Saunders Co., 1982.)

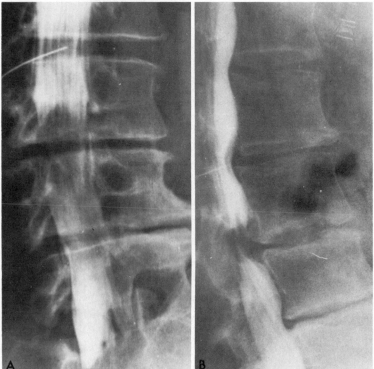

Figure 2–28. Metrizamide myelogram reveals a complete block at the L3–4 level due to spinal stenosis. *A,* In the anteroposterior view note the block centered at the disc space with a paintbrush appearance. *B,* In the lateral view note that the compression is both anterior and posterior, is extradural in appearance, and is centered at the level of the disc space. (From Rothman, R. H., and Simeone, F. A.: The Spine, 2nd ed. Philadelphia, W. B. Saunders Co., 1982.)

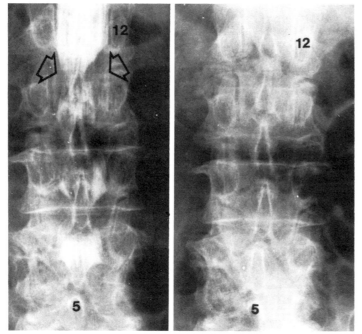

Figure 2–29. This metrizamide myelogram illustrates severe spinal stenosis from L1 to the sacrum. Note the enlarged facet joints, narrowing of the anterior laminar spaces, and tapering of the dye column at T12–L1. (From Rothman, R. H., and Simeone, F. A.: The Spine, 2nd ed. Philadelphia, W. B. Saunders Co., 1982.)

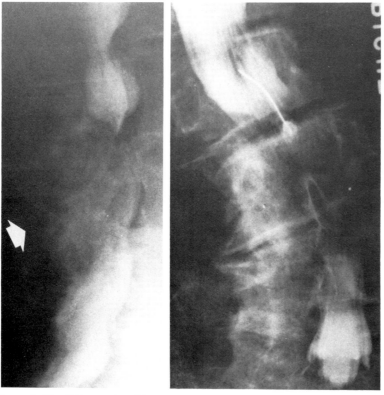

Figure 2–30. This metrizamide myelogram illustrates a complete block due to spinal stenosis at the L3–4 level. A lumbar scoliosis is present with lateral spondylolisthesis, disc degeneration, and decompensation of the facet joints. (From Rothman, R. H., and Simeone, F. A.: The Spine, 2nd ed. Philadelphia, W. B. Saunders Co., 1982.)

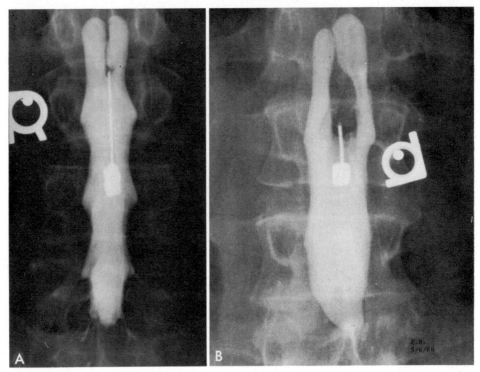

Figure 2–31. *A,* This oil myelographic defect is from the spinal needle itself. In this case it is small and symmetrical. *B,* A more dramatic needle defect which is larger and less symmetrical. (From Rothman, R. H., and Simeone, F. A.: The Spine, 2nd ed. Philadelphia, W. B. Saunders Co., 1982.)

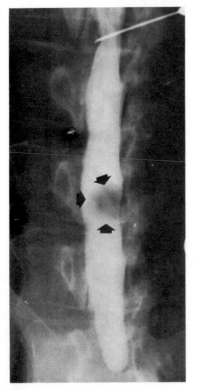

Figure 2–32. This myelographic defect represents a small extradural hematoma produced from a previous puncture. (From Rothman, R. H., and Simeone, F. A.: The Spine, 2nd ed. Philadelphia, W. B. Saunders Co., 1982.)

needle can vary tremendously in size and occasionally is so dramatic as to mimic a space-occupying lesion (Fig. 2–31). Similarly, an epidural hematoma resulting from a spinal needle advanced too far anteriorly can produce a defect compatible with an epidural mass (Fig. 2–32). For this reason, the spinal puncture should be performed at a level well away from the expected site of disc herniation. The usual puncture site is the L2–L3 level, unless a high lumbar disc is suspected.

Artifacts are also commonly seen in individuals who have previously had oil contrast media myelography, particularly in the presence of previous surgery. Picard and others[37] reviewed 1950 studies and demonstrated an incidence of "scarring" in 14 per cent of patients who did not have surgery and in 47 per cent of those who were subjected to operative intervention. (The preference for the descriptive term "scarring" versus the anatomic terms of arachnoiditis and epiduritis prevents confusion and controversy (Fig. 2–33). Although the occurrence of epidural lesions without previous surgery is rare, there are a myriad of possible postsurgery and post–previous myelogram artifacts that can very easily obscure or mimic new pathologic conditions.

In conclusion, although it is appreciated that the myelogram is at least

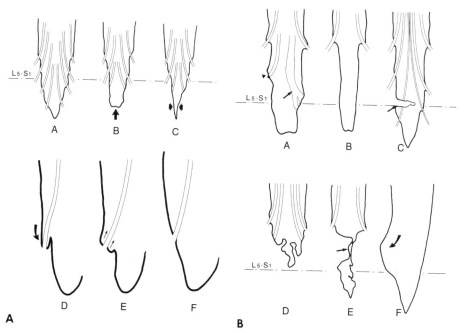

Figure 2–33. *A,* Arachnoid scarring. Stage 1. (a) Diagram of normal appearances. (b) Short and blunted theca. (c) Narrowed, filiform cul-de-sac — lesions of the nerve roots. (d) Vertical position of the nerve roots and approximation to the theca. (e) Retraction of the subarachnoid extensions above and below the nerve root, giving a "stump" appearance. (f) Total effacement of the root sheath. *B,* Arachnoid scarring. Stage 2. (a) Shortening of the theca; lesions above L5–S1. "Enlarged roots" (arrow). Stump-like root sheath (arrowhead). (b) Tubular appearance. The root sheaths are completely obliterated. Epidural lesions. (c) Characteristic "pinched" appearance. Mixed arachnoid and epidural lesions. (d) Ragged lower end to an amputated theca. (e) Persistent stenosis — postoperative meningocele. (From Picard, L., Roland, J., Blanchot, P., David, R., et al.: Scarring of the theca and the nerve roots as seen in radiculography. J. Neuroradiol., *4*:29, 1977.)

90 per cent accurate, with both false positive and false negative results, it still remains extremely helpful and essential as a diagnostic tool in the pre-operative evaluation of the patient with a suspected herniated disc. Myelography should not be used in patients who are not surgical candidates to substantiate or disprove legal claims, nor should it be used as the primary factor in deciding whether or not a particular patient should undergo surgical intervention. There are other invasive studies (mentioned in the following section) that can help to verify the surgeon's suspicions. A patient with a classic history of a disc herniation with a clear-cut neurologic deficit and a positive straight leg raising test who has not responded to nonoperative treatment should not be denied surgery simply on the basis of an equivocal or negative myelogram. Fortunately, this is a rare phenomenon.

DISCOGRAPHY

Discography has not proved to be essential or reliable in our experience and that of others.[9, 28] It is performed by placing a fine-gauge spinal needle into a disc space under image intensification, either posterolaterally or transdiscally. Radiopaque dye is injected into the interspace, and information is recorded regarding the amount of dye accepted, the pressure necessary to inject the material, the configuration of the opaque material, and the reproduction of the patient's pain. The diagnostic potential in the *lumbar* spine, therefore, is realized by the clinical response of the patient, the resistance of the disc to infusion, and the roentgenographic appearance of the disc. A normal discogram may be helpful in ruling out disc degeneration, but abnormalities compatible with a diagnosis of multiple degenerative discs are so common, particularly with increasing age,[36] that little significance can be given to an abnormal discogram in terms of localizing the source of a patient's pain. Even though one might reliably reproduce the patient's spinal pain with a discogenic study, the results of spinal surgery for relief of back pain alone without herniations caused by degenerative disc disease are disappointing.[47] Discography, however, may be most helpful when spine fusion is being contemplated, particularly in the geriatric population with scoliosis, since one may lengthen the course of the fusion *if* the intended limits are associated roentgenographically with significant disc space degeneration or true subclinical herniation.[46]

The study is essential in chymopapain therapy and may be helpful in documentation of significant lateral disc herniations not appreciated on myelography. It is our feeling, however, that in most cases the study is not essential, particularly in light of the diagnostic sensitivity afforded by water-soluble contrast myelography, epidural venography, and computerized axial tomography. Our feelings are the same concerning nerve root sleeve injections, which can be particularly unpleasant for the patient if the nerve, rather than the sheath, is violated by the introduced needle tip.

EPIDURAL VENOGRAPHY

It is possible to visualize the epidural venous plexus by the insertion of a large-gauge needle into the marrow of the lumbar spinous process with the subsequent injection of angiographic contrast material. In 1961, Shobinger, Kringer, and Soble[44] used the technique to demonstrate intervertebral disc herniations and certain intraspinous tumors. As a result of patient discomfort and less than ideal perfusions, catheterization of the iliac veins with sacrolumbar venous visualization was performed and reported by Helander and Lindbom in 1955.[26] Bücheler and Janson in 1973,[7] LePage in 1974,[30] and Gargano and others in 1974[18] improved the technique and provided better visualization of the epidural veins by selected catheterization of the ascending lumbar veins.

The vertebral venous system can be divided into three major components. The first is the interosseous system, which is of no diagnostic value at this point in time. The second network is composed of the anterior internal vertebral vein and the ascending external vertebral vein, the emissary or radicular veins, and the posterior intervertebral veins. All but the last-mentioned veins are of diagnostic importance as far as mass lesions within the spinal canal are concerned. The third component is the external vertebral vein system, particularly the ascending lumbar and lateral sacral veins, which allow access to the previously mentioned second venous network (see Fig. 1–19).

The concepts and facts that justify utilization of this well-tolerated but invasive technique are as follows:

1. There should be a consistent and reliable epidural venous system in proximity to the anterior limits of the spinal canal and neural foramina. The variations in venous anatomy usually affect the number and caliber of the veins rather than their location within the confines of the spinal canal.

2. Since the easily compressible veins traverse the spinal canal in proximity to susceptible neural structures, abnormal venous filling can indirectly imply mass effect with encroachment.

3. As a result of the capacious anatomy of the spine at L4–L5 and particularly at L5–S1 and the limited subarachnoid extensions along the spinal nerves, an ancillary study that can provide more sensitivity (fewer false negatives) than the myelogram should be available. This is particularly true when the myelogram is equivocal in the presence of hard neurologic findings and tension signs.

Several authors[18, 20, 31, 32] have demonstrated that there is greater sensitivity with epidural venography than with oil-based myelography, particularly in the capacious L5–S1 segment. In the absence of previous surgery and in the presence of adequate filling, the following abnormalities (modified from Gargano[18] and Theron[50]) are felt to be compatible with disc herniations and other anatomic changes resulting in spinal canal compromise:

1. Unilateral or bilateral complete or partial interruption of the anterior internal or anterior external vertebral veins.

2. Increased contrast accumulation or enlargement of the anterior

internal or anterior external vertebral vein above, below, or continuous with the herniation secondary to venous stasis or bypass phenomenon.

3. Deviation of the anterior vertebral veins without cessation of venous flow.

4. Deviation or occlusion of the emissary or radicular veins accompanying the spinal vein that is indicative of lateral herniation or lateral encroachment (Figs. 2–34 to 2–40).

To avoid inadequate venous filling that would present problems with reliable interpretation, patients are considered candidates for study if they have not had any previous lumbar spinal surgery. Furthermore, to avoid iatrogenic artifacts (particularly of retrograde filling), bilateral trans-femoral catheterization is performed, using the ascending lumbar vein on the one side and the anterior lateral sacral vein on the contralateral side. We consider a significant dye allergy and a previous history of thrombophlebitis to be absolute contraindications to epidural venography. This study has been well tolerated by our patients; one case of nonlethal pulmonary embolus in over 100 cases has been the authors' only significant complication.

The authors use this study primarily when myelography has been either equivocal or negative despite hard neurologic findings or positive tension signs. It is important to realize that this study has not supplanted

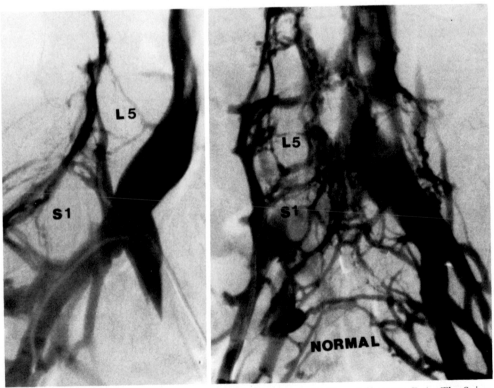

Figure 2–34. Normal epidural venogram. (From Rothman, R. H., and Simeone, F. A.: The Spine, 2nd ed. Philadelphia, W. B. Saunders Co., 1982.)

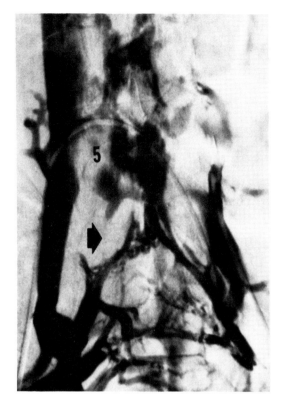

Figure 2–35. Epidural venogram illustrates obliteration of the anterior internal vertebral vein at the L5–S1 level unilaterally. Lateral disc herniation was noted at this location. (From Rothman, R. H., and Simeone, F. A.: The Spine, 2nd ed. Philadelphia, W. B. Saunders Co., 1982.)

myelography but rather, when used in conjunction, has increased the precision of our diagnostic capabilities. The myelogram is still considered essential for localization and definition of subarachnoid space compromise and mass lesion. Although metrizamide may eventually obviate the need for epidural venography in the near future, the fourth generation CAT scan may eventually do the same for myelography.

COMPUTERIZED AXIAL TOMOGRAPHY

Fourth generation computerized axial tomography (CAT) represents a most sophisticated, relatively new noninvasive diagnostic modality that can pictorially quantify dimensions of the spinal canal and neural foramina and define by varying tissue densities the source of neurovascular compromise (Fig. 2–41).

This scanning delivers a radiation exposure of from one to three rads for an entire exam, which, although not significantly greater than the exposure from GI studies or angiography, is more than that resulting from plain roentgenography and therefore should be selectively utilized.

CAT scanning can be used in localizing and defining the extent of the traumatic, infectious, or neoplastic involvement of the axial skeleton in cases of back pain without severe neural involvement in conjunction with laboratory data such as a Ca/P level, alkaline phosphatase level, sedimen-

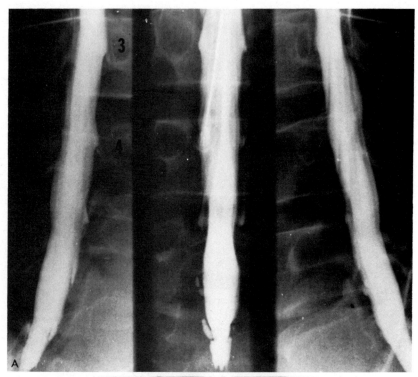

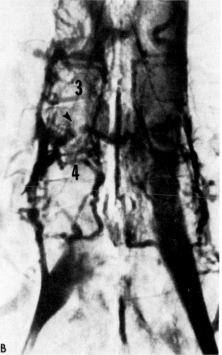

Figure 2–36. This patient had unremitting L4 nerve root symptoms. *A*, This oil myelogram was completely normal. *B*, The epidural venogram revealed a defect in the radicular vein at the L3–L4 level. A free disc fragment found in the foramen well laterally was the source of nerve root compression. (From Rothman, R. H., and Simeone, F. A.: The Spine, 2nd ed. Philadelphia, W. B. Saunders Co., 1982.)

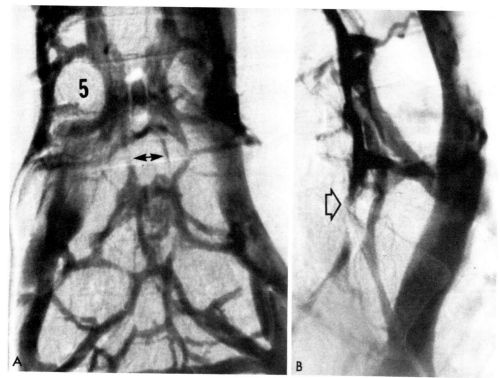

Figure 2–37. Epidural venogram reveals occlusion of the anterior internal vertebral veins bilaterally at L5–S1 due to a central disc herniation as seen in the anteroposterior view *(A)* and in the lateral view *(B)*. (From Rothman, R. H., and Simeone, F. A.: The Spine, 2nd ed. Philadelphia, W. B. Saunders Co., 1982.)

Figure 2–38. This epidural venogram illustrates interruption of the anterior intervertebral vein at L5–S1 on the right. This patient had unremitting right sciatica and a normal oil myelogram. (From Rothman, R. H., and Simeone, F. A.: The Spine, 2nd ed. Philadelphia, W. B. Saunders Co., 1982.)

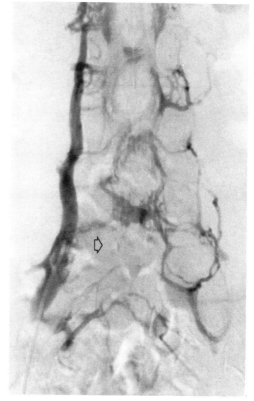

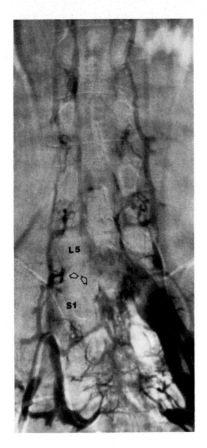

Figure 2–39. This epidural venogram reveals obliteration of the anterior intervertebral vein at L5–S1 associated with obliteration of the radicular vein at the same level. This patient had a large lateral disc herniation at L5–S1 compatible with this defect. (From Rothman, R. H., and Simeone, F. A.: The Spine, 2nd ed. Philadelphia, W. B. Saunders Co., 1982.)

Figure 2–40. This epidural venogram reveals obliteration of the anterior internal vertebral vein and radicular vein at both L4–5 and L5–S1 secondary to narrowing of the lateral recess. (From Rothman, R. H., and Simeone, F. A.: The Spine, 2nd ed. Philadelphia, W. B. Saunders Co., 1982.)

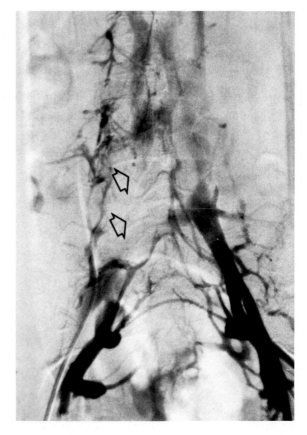

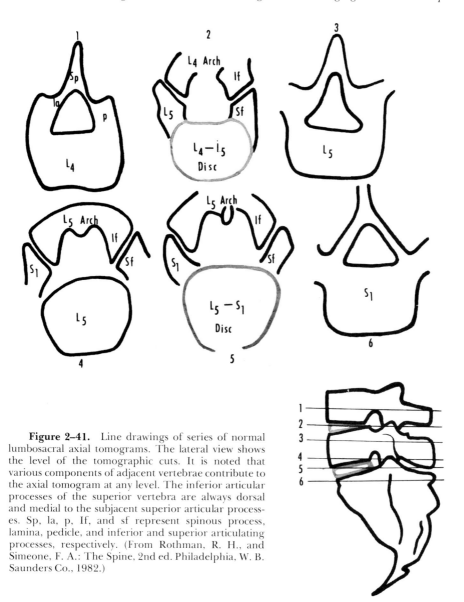

Figure 2–41. Line drawings of series of normal lumbosacral axial tomograms. The lateral view shows the level of the tomographic cuts. It is noted that various components of adjacent vertebrae contribute to the axial tomogram at any level. The inferior articular processes of the superior vertebra are always dorsal and medial to the subjacent superior articular processes. Sp, la, p, If, and sf represent spinous process, lamina, pedicle, and inferior and superior articulating processes, respectively. (From Rothman, R. H., and Simeone, F. A.: The Spine, 2nd ed. Philadelphia, W. B. Saunders Co., 1982.)

tation rate, and protein electrophoresis. It is particularly helpful when technetium or gallium bone scanning or plain film tomography has already localized the site of pathology.[17, 19, 45]

In the clinical syndrome of lumbar disc disease, the intimate relationship of the theca and the nerve roots to the annulus and foraminal canal delineated by the CAT scan can allow the clinician to define what components, if any, are compromising the neural elements. The full spectrum of the aging phenomenon that affects the spine can be documented from the simple isolated disc protrusion in a relatively normal canal in an individual in the younger age group to the spinal canal and foramina compromised by facet and laminar hypertrophy, annular bulging, and liga-

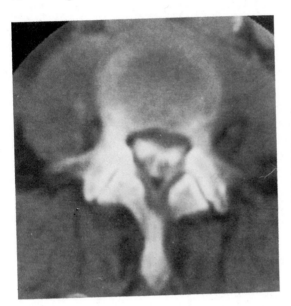

Figure 2–42. A metrizamide-enhanced computerized axial tomogram showing a soft tissue density compromising the ventral border of the theca, a true central disc herniation. Also note the excellent definition of the facet joints, the outline of the ligamentum flavum, and the relatively black presentation of epidural fat. (Courtesy of M. Judith Donovan-Post, M.D., University of Miami, Miami, Florida.)

mentum flavum redundancy and hypertrophy, i.e., spinal stenosis, in the older population group. The ability of the computer to differentiate bone from ligament from disc and fat and neural tissue allows one to define the extent as well as the location of the neural compromise. This is particularly true in cases in which metrizamide is used to enhance tissue differentiation (Figs. 2–42, 2–43).

The clinician can subsequently define the pathology as well as plan the appropriate operative approach. As with myelography, however, CAT scanning should be a preoperative study that confirms the clinical impression already substantiated by objective neurologic deficit (motor and reflex asymmetry) and positive tension signs (straight leg raising for sciatic root,

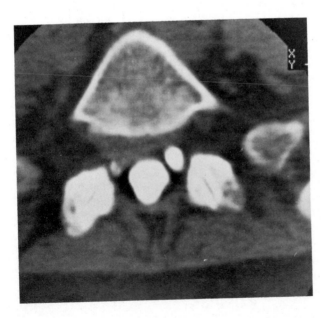

Figure 2–43. Another metrizamide-enhanced computerized tomogram at the lumbosacral junction. One can clearly see the soft tissue compromise of the white-enhanced nerve root. Also note that this patient has had previous surgery and there is no lamina or spinous process. (Courtesy of M. Judith Donovan-Post, M.D., University of Miami, Miami, Florida.)

femoral stretch for upper and midlumbar roots, and prolonged lumbar extension or stress ambulation for intermittent neurogenic claudication).

Although a CSF protein analysis is not a standard part of CAT scanning, the study (when performed well) can obviate myelographic definition in many straightforward cases.[39] When there is ambiguity, enhancement meylography or epidural venography can provide data that would virtually eliminate false positive and false negative interpretations.

ELECTROMYOGRAPHY

Electromyography documents the functional integrity of the motor unit, that is, the anterior horn cell, the axon, the neuromuscular junctions, and the muscle fibers involved. When muscle groups of either anterior or posterior rami innervation demonstrate abnormal irritability (fibrillations), abnormally large motor unit action potentials, or an increased number of polyphasic motor unit action potentials on electromyography, abnormal acute or chronic neurofunction is implied.

Electromyography, however, does not define the altered anatomy causing the neural dysfunction. The diagnostic specificity and sensitivity realized with the combination of a well-performed physical examination, epidural venography, water-soluble myelography, or CAT scan has obviated the authors' use of electromyography in the diagnosis of symptomatic lumbar disc disease.

However, when there is a suspicion of metabolic, ischemic, or heredofamilial peripheral neuropathies, the electromyogram can be diagnostically helpful.

THE DIFFERENTIAL SPINAL BLOCK

Differential spinal anesthesia, as described by Ahlgren,[1] involves the serial injection of increasing concentrations of an anesthetic into the subarachnoid space. On occasion, this has proved to be helpful in differentiating between organic and functional pain and is particularly useful in patients with serious emotional problems, in patients with a paucity of objective findings, in the presence of severe pain, and in patients who are suspected of malingering.[45]

Subarachnoid tap is performed utilizing a 20-gauge needle with the patient in the lateral recumbent position with the painful leg side down. Injections are made at 10 minute intervals of 5 ml. of isotonic saline (placebo), 10 ml. of 0.2% procaine (sympathetic block), 10 ml. of 0.5 procaine (sensory block), and 10 ml. of 1% procaine (motor block). After each injection, the patient is asked to evaluate his pain at rest and after a passive manipulation such as the straight leg raising test. Evaluation of vasomotor sensory and motor function is also conducted to determine the efficacy of the anesthetic.

With the use of this test, the etiology of the pain can usually be ascribed to *primarily* an organic lesion or to a functional basis. It is also possible to determine if the organic pain is mediated principally by the sensory or sympathetic portion of the nervous system.

The results are most dramatic when the patient is either completely relieved of pain with only saline or experiences no relief with 1% procaine, or when the procaine produces motor paralysis or a sensory level several dermatomes above the pain site. In both of these circumstances, the etiology of the pain can be interpreted as nonorganic or primarily functional in nature.

REFERENCES

1. Ahlgren, E. W., et al.: Diagnosis of pain with a graduated spinal block technique. JAMA, *195*:125, 1966.
2. Allbrook, D.: Movements of the lumbar spinal column. J. Bone Joint Surg., *39B*:339, 1957.
3. Baker, R., Hillman, B. J., McLennan, J. E., et al.: Sequelae of metrizamide myelography in 200 examinations. Am. J. Roentgenol., *139*:499, 1978.
4. Bentson, J. R.: Comparison of metrizamide with other myelographic agents. Clin. Orthop., *127*:111, 1977.
5. Bernini, P. M., Wiesel, S., and Rothman, R.: Metrizamide myelography and the identification of anomalous lumbosacral nerve root. J. Bone Joint Surg., *62A*:1203, 1980.
6. Bernini, P. M., Floeman, Y., Marvel, J., and Rothman, R.: Multiple thoracic spine fractures complicating ankylosing hyperostosis of the spine. J. Trauma. In press, 1981.
7. Bücheler, E., and Janson, R.: Combined catheter venography of the lumbar venous system and the inferior vena cava. Br. J. Radiol., *46*:655, 1973.
8. DePalma, A., and Rothman, R.: Surgery of the lumbar spine. Clin. Orthop., *63*:162, 1969.
9. DePalma, A., and Rothman, R.: The Intervertebral Disc. Philadelphia, W. B. Saunders Co., 1970.
10. Edeiken, J., and Pitt, M. J.: The radiologic diagnosis of disc disease. Orthop. Clin. North Am., *2(2)*:405, 1971.
11. Ericksen, M. F.: Some aspects of aging in the lumbar spine. Am. J. Phys. Anthropol., *45*:575, 1976.
12. Ericksen, M. F.: Aging in the lumbar spine (L1 and L2). Am. J. Phys. Anthropol., *48*:241, 1978.
13. Edgar, M. A., and Park, W. M.: Induced pain patterns on passive straight leg raising in lower lumbar disc protrusion. J. Bone Joint Surg., *56B*:658, 1974.
14. Farfan, H. F., Osteria, V., and Lamy, C.: The mechanical etiology of spondylolysis and spondylolisthesis. Clin. Orthop., *117*:40, 1976.
15. Fitzgerald, J. A. W., and Newman, P. H.: Degenerative spondylolisthesis. J. Bone Joint Surg., *58B*:184, 1976.
16. Ford, L. T., Gilula, L. A., Murphy, W. A., and Gado, M.: Analysis of gas in vacuum lumbar disc. Am. J. Roentgenol., *128*:1056, 1977.
17. Gargano, F. P., Jacobson, R. E., and Rosomoff, H.: Transverse axial tomography of the spine. Neuroradiology, *6*:254, 1974.
18. Gargano, F. P., Meyer, J. D., and Sheldon, J. J.: Transfemoral ascending lumbar catheterization of the epidural veins in lumbar disk disease. Radiology, *111*:329, 1974.
19. Gargano, F. P.: Transverse axial tomography of the spine. Crit. Rev. Clin. Radiol. Nucl. Med., *8(3)*:279, 1976.
20. Gershater, R., and St. Louis, E. L.: Lumbar epidural venography. Radiology, *131*:409, 1979.
21. Ghelman, B., and Freiberger, R. H.: The limbus vertebra: an anterior disc herniation demonstrated by discography. Am. J. Roentgenol., *127*:854, 1976.
22. Gonsette, R.: An experimental and clinical assessment of water-soluble contrast medium in neuroradiology: a new medium-dimer-X. Clin. Radiol., *22*:44, 1971.
23. Grainger, R. G., Kendall, B. E., and Wylie, I. G.: Lumbar myelography with metrizamide — a new nonionic contrast medium. Br. J. Radiol., *49*:996, 1976.

24. Hakelius, A., and Hindmarsh, J.: The comparative reliability of preoperative diagnostic methods in lumbar disc surgery. Acta Orthop. Scand., *43*:234, 1972.
25. Harris, R., and Macnab, I.: Structural changes in the lumbar intervertebral discs. J. Bone Joint Surg., *35B*:304, 1954.
26. Helander, C. G., and Lindbom, A.: Sacrolumbar venography. Acta Radiol., *44*:410, 1955.
27. Hilton, R. C., Ball, J., and Benn, R. T.: Vertebral end-plate lesions (Schmorl's nodes) in the dorsolumbar spine. Ann. Rheumatol., *35*:127, 1976.
28. Holt, E.: The question of lumbar discography. J. Bone Joint Surg., *50*:720, 1968.
29. LaRocca, H., and Macnab, I.: Value of pre-employment radiography assessment of the lumbar spine. R. Ind. Med., *39(6)*:253, 1970.
30. LePage, J. R.: Transfemoral ascending lumbar catheterization of the epidural veins. Radiology, *111*:337, 1974.
31. MacNab, I., St. Louis, E. L., Grabias, S. L., et al.: Selective ascending lumbosacral venography in the assessment of the lumbar disc herniation. J. Bone Joint Surg., *58A*:1093, 1976.
32. MacNab, I.: Backache. Baltimore, Williams & Wilkins Co., 1977.
33. Magnussen, W.: Uber die bedingungen des herrortretens der werkluken gelenkspatte auf dem rontgenbilde. Acta Radiol., *18*:733, 1937.
34. Magora, A., and Schwartz, A.: Relation between the low back pain syndrome and x-ray findings. Scand. J. Rehabil. Med., *8*:115, 1976.
35. O'Dell, C. W., Coel, M. N., and Igelzi, R. J.: Ascending lumbar venography in lumbar disc disease. J. Bone Joint Surg., *59A*:159, 1977.
36. Patrick, B. S.: Lumbar discography. A five year study. Surg. Neurol., *1*:267, 1973.
37. Picard, L., et al.: Scarring of the theca. Neuroradiology, *4(1)*:29, 1977.
38. Posner, I., White, A., Edwards, W. T., and Hayes, W. C.: Assessment of clinical stability of the lumbar and lumbosacral spine. Presented Eastern Orthopedic Association, Oct. 15–19, 1980.
39. Post, M. J., Gargano, F. P., Vining, D. Q., and Rosomoff, H. L.: A comparison of radiographic methods of diagnosing constrictive lesions of the spinal canal. J. Neurosurg., *48*:360, 1978.
40. Ratheke, L.: Uber kalkablagerungen in den zwischenwirbelscheiben. Forgschr. Roint. Genstr., 45, 1932.
41. Resnick, D., and Niwayama, G.: Intervertebral disk herniations: cartilaginous (Schmorl's) nodes. Radiology, *126*:57, 1978.
42. Roland, J., Treil, J., Larde, D., et al.: Lumbar phlebography in the diagnosis of disc herniations. J. Neurosurg., *49*:544, 1978.
43. Schmorl, G., and Jungham, H.: The Human Spine in Health and Diseases. New York, Grune and Stratton, 1971.
44. Schobinger, R. A., Krueger, E., and Sobel, G.: Comparison of intraosseous vertebral venography and pantopaque myelography in the diagnosis of surgical conditions of the lumbar spine and nerve roots. Radiology, *77*:397, 1961.
45. Sheldon, J. J., Sersland, T., and Leborgne, J.: Computed tomography of the lower lumbar vertebral column. Radiology, *124*:113, 1977.
46. Simmons, E. H., and Segil, C. M.: An evaluation of discography in the localization of symptomatic level in discogenic disease of the spine. Clin. Orthop., *108*:57, 1975.
47. Spangfort, E. V.: The lumbar disc herniation. A computer-aided analysis of 2504 operations. Acta Orthop. Scand., *142* (Suppl.) 61, 1972.
48. Symposium: Lumbar arachnoiditis: nomenclature, etiology and pathology. Spine, *3(1)*:21, 1978.
49. Taillard, W.: Etiology of spondylolisthesis. Clin. Orthop., *117*:30, 1976.
50. Theron, J., Houtteville, J. P., Ammerich, H., et al.: Lumbar phlebography by catheterization of the lateral sacral and ascending lumbar veins with abdominal compression. Neuroradiology, *11*:175, 1976.
51. Torgerson, W. R., and Dotter, W. E.: Comparative roentgenographic study of the asymptomatic and symptomatic lumbar spine. J. Bone Joint Surg., *58A*:850, 1976.
52. Vernon-Roberts, B., and Pirie, C. J.: Degenerative changes in the intervertebral discs of the lumbar spine and their sequelae. Rheumatol. Rehabil., *16*:13, 1977.
53. Wiesel, S., Ignatius, P., Marvel, J. P., et al.: Intradural neurofibroma stimulating lumbar disc disease. J. Bone Joint Surg., *58A*:1040, 1976.
54. Wigh, R., and Anthony, H.: Transitional lumbosacral discs: probability of herniation. Spine, *6(2)*:168, 1981.

Chapter 3

CLINICAL SYNDROMES

INTRODUCTION

Degeneration of the lumbar disc and the associated phenomenon of degenerative arthritis of the facet joints are the most common causes of low back and leg pain. The syndromes that evolve are multifaceted and must be recognized as such if the diagnoses are to be correct and the treatments effective. One sees with disturbing regularity missed diagnoses of herniated lumbar discs that present in an atypical fashion, unfamiliar to the practitioner. It is equally precarious, however, to polarize one's thinking at the opposite extreme and attribute all cases of back and leg pain to abnormalities of the intervertebral disc. A wide spectrum of vascular, infectious, and neoplastic lesions can mimic the herniated lumbar disc. In this section, the authors will attempt to outline the classic pictures of lumbar disc degeneration, as well as the more common variants.

It is important from the outset to recognize that the clinical syndromes to be discussed represent manifestations of the sequential spectrum of degeneration that affects the "three joint complex."[14] The clinical presentation will range from backache, with and without referred pain, to radicular pain to neurogenic claudication. These symptoms are a reflection of the totality of degeneration of the intervertebral discs and the facet joints. Furthermore, symptoms can be conveyed over well-defined, frequently simultaneously stimulated pain pathways. These include the sinovertebral nerves to the annulus and theca, the spinal nerves, and the medial and lateral branches of the posterior rami. Systemic analysis of these pathways will allow for a more exact therapeutic solution.

HISTORY

Back Pain

The majority of patients with degenerative disc disease in the lumbar spine have low back pain as the earliest symptom. Spangfort's computerized analysis of 2504 disc operations demonstrated a mean duration of low back pain of 5.6 years prior to surgery, and this temporal disability preceded the onset of leg complaints by nearly two years.[39] Weber's[43] excellent prospective study of lumbar disc herniation suggested that in more than 90 per cent of patients studied, there were nearly ten years of episodic low back pain prior to the insidious onset of a radicular component. The patient recalls that after periods of demanding physical activity or of seemingly benign but prolonged postures, pain appears in the lumbosacral area. The pain may last a few days and usually subsides with limitation of activity and bed rest. The pain pattern at this time is mechanical in nature, in the sense that it is made worse by standing, lifting, and prolonged sitting and is relieved by rest.

It is the authors' feeling that pain at this stage is caused by early degeneration of the annulus fibrosus and desiccation of the nucleus pulposus. Since the nucleus no longer functions as a perfect gel with viscoelastic properties, it will therefore transmit forces in a nonlinear and asymmetric fashion[23] (Fig. 3–1). These intermittent episodes of mechanical low back pain are nonspecific and cannot, in fact, be differentiated from the syndromes commonly characterized as "low back sprain," "muscular strain," or "acute lumbago." Because these syndromes frequently progress to the more typical disc hernia with unequivocal findings, we feel that by implication, the pathologic cause for these episodes of low back pain is disc degeneration.

Since the disc has dorsally situated sinovertebral sensory nerves,

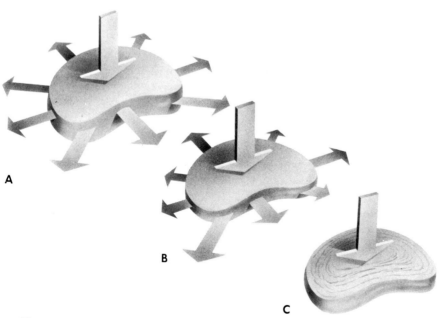

Figure 3–1. Distribution of forces in the normal and abnormal disc. *A,* When the disc functions normally, as in the early decades of life, the nucleus distributes the forces of compression and tension equally to all parts of the annulus. *B,* With degeneration, the nucleus no longer functions as a perfect gel and the forces transmitted to the annulus are unequal. *C,* With advanced degeneration of the nucleus, the distribution of forces to the annulus from within is completely lost since the nucleus now acts as a solid rather than a liquid. For this reason, disc herniation is unusual in the elderly. (From Rothman, R. H., and Simeone, F. A.: The Spine, 2nd ed. Philadelphia, W. B. Saunders Co., 1982.)

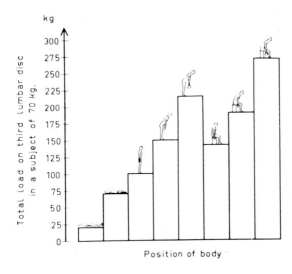

Figure 3–2. This figure illustrates the total load on the third lumbar disc in a subject weighing 70 kg. (From Nachemson, A.: In vivo discometry in lumbar discs with irregular nucleograms. Acta Orthop. Scand. 36:426, 1965.)

degeneration can reasonably be implicated in this pain syndrome. The initial age of onset of low back pain, usually the late twenties and early thirties, coincides with the obliteration of the vascular supply to the nucleus pulposus and all but the most peripheral aspects of the annulus fibrosus. The subsequent age-related defective defusion mechanism at the vertebral end-plate-annular interface[8, 27] provides a basis for the loss of structural integrity of the disc at this time in the aging process of the axial skeleton. The mechanical intensification and relief seen in this clinical syndrome can also be attributed to disc degeneration and are easily understood in light of Nachemson's[31, 32] landmark in vivo determination of disc pressure in various postures (Fig. 3–2).

It should be re-emphasized that at this early stage, disc degeneration cannot be clearly differentiated from certain other common causes of low back pain, such as neural arch defects, postural strain, and unstable lumbosacral mechanisms.

With the passage of time, these episodes may become more frequent and intense and may lead to more disability. Between acute episodes of back pain, the patient usually describes a sense of stiffness, weakness, or instability that is present at a low but noticeable level. These symptoms are probably manifestations of abnormal motion segment (vertebral body, disc, and facet joint) behavior alterations, which Kulack and others[23] have appreciated in their mathematical and two-dimensional finite element models. These defined changes occur in disc geometry and annular structural integrity and in the way the disc nucleus is pressurized prior to load. Discogenic pain usually has the definite mechanical quality of being accentuated with prolonged sitting and standing. There is a clinical correlation of increased symptoms with increased load. Pain that increases while the patient is in bed at night is more suggestive of a neoplastic process or infection. The pain of disc disease is characteristically intermittent, and one should be wary when the patient states that from the onset the pain has been unrelenting and progressive, as in infectious or neoplastic states.

Injury is frequently noted by the patient at some time during the

Experimental flow of fluid in autopsy discs.

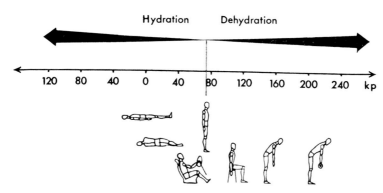

Figure 3–3. Theoretical calculation on the hydration-dehydration points as obtained experimentally by Kramer combined with the findings of intradiscal pressure measurements by Nachemson. (From Nachemson, A.: Toward a better understanding of low-back pain: A review of the mechanics of the lumbar disc. Rheumatol. Rehabil., *14*(3):129, 1975.)

clinical course, and in many instances, spine pain was present to a greater or lesser degree prior to injury. Weber's[43] study revealed precipitating events for the first episode of low back pain in 55 per cent of patients who eventually developed disc herniations. The trauma that was reported, however, ranged from a falling episode to lifting and heavy work activity to nothing more serious than an abrupt movement. It is interesting that these incidents usually occur during the early hours of the day after the patient has had an extended supine position in sleep, when the turgor (function of increased hydration) of the nucleus pulposus is at its maximum[32] (Fig. 3–3).

Our current concepts of the pathophysiologic features of symptomatic disc disease show trauma to be a precipitating rather than a causative factor. Jayson and others[19] subjected 78 cadaver intervertebral discs to discography and roentgenographically classified their nuclear morphology. When the discs were subjected to compressive loads, bursting most commonly occurred into the adjacent vertebral bodies and not posteriorly. When there was nuclear herniation posterolaterally and directly posterior, it occurred in discs that were previously noted to have posterolateral, direct posterior, or degenerative nuclear morphology. Although the discs were subjected to compressive forces only, the importance of the premorbid nuclear and annular status is obvious.

Excessive stress applied to a young, healthy spine will fracture the osseous elements of the vertebra before the disc is ruptured. When disc herniation occurs in young, healthy spines not yet affected by disc degeneration, it is likely that the herniation will follow areas of premorbid structural weakness, namely, the residual indentations in the cartilaginous end-plate that are left as a result of notochord or embryologic vascular regression, yielding Schmorl's nodes.[36] The other premorbid area of relative structural weakness persists at the interface between the cartilaginous end-plate and the ossified portion of the vertebral body. Keller[21] reported two cases of adolescents with disc and vertebral rim prolapse with significant spinal canal compromise and symptoms, confirmed by myelography.

Referred Pain

When certain mesodermal structures, such as ligaments, periosteum, joint capsule, and the annulus, are subjected to abnormal stimuli such as excessive stretching or the injection of hypertonic saline, a deep, ill-defined, dull, aching discomfort is noted that may be referred into the areas of the lumbosacral joint, sacroiliac joint, and the buttocks, as well as the legs[22, 29] (Fig. 3–4). The pattern of referral is to the area designated the sclerotome, which has the same embryonic origin as the mesodermal tissues stimulated. Although this peripheral pathway can explain the referred pattern, the significant individual variations that are encountered necessitate the consideration of central neural pathways. Indeed, Kellgren[22] has concluded that the referred distribution of pain depends not only on segmental innervation, but also on the severity of pain and the extent to which an individual is cognizant of the stimulated components of the axial skeleton.

Pain of this type can often present concurrently with radicular pain from nerve root tension. The deeper, boring pain is classically attributed to distribution along the myotome and sclerotomes, and the sharper and better localized superficial pain is conveyed via the dermatomes[10]; the two may be easily confused. Moreover, sympathetic dystrophic signs and

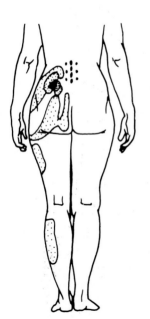

NORMAL

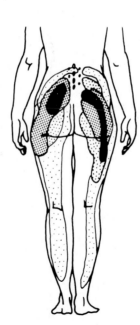

ABNORMAL

Figure 3–4. Pain referral pattern for asymptomatic and symptomatic subjects. This confirms that the pain referral pattern from stimulation of the lumbar facet joint is in the typical locations of lumbago. (From Mooney, V., and Robertson, J.: The facet syndrome. Clin. Orthop. *115*:149, 1976.)

symptoms caused by nerve root encroachment can further confuse the presentation, since the causalgia may exist with or without the more classic complaints associated with radiculopathy.[3] Thus, it is clear that not all leg pain is a result of nerve root compression per se.

Radicular Symptoms

Pressure on an inflamed nerve root by a disc fragment, bulging annulus, or compromised lateral recess may produce pain and motor or sensory signs and symptoms in the lower extremities. It had been first suggested by Smyth and Wright in 1958[40] and was later demonstrated by MacNab[25] that normal nerve roots subjected to compression will produce paresthesias, whereas nerves that are inflamed will yield a painful response to manipulation.

The etiologic role of mechanical tension on the nerve root yielding radicular pain is generally accepted, but whether there is damage to the intrinsic structure of the neural tissue or its accompanying vasculature or both is uncertain.[30] The production of pain with straight leg raising or cross leg raising for the L5 and S1 spinal nerves and reverse straight leg raising for an L4 radiculopathy reflects the mechanical inability of the nerve root to yield to tension in and around the neural foramina.

The inflammatory component of the radicular syndrome is also of significance, but again, the causative agents are uncertain. With the evolution of annular rents, the avascular nucleus pulposus may evoke an autoimmune response and act as a causative factor. This conclusion has been theorized owing to the susceptibility of the nerve roots to inflammatory agents and an enhanced immune cellular response to homogenized disc material in both animals and humans.[5, 12] Furthermore, a contributory humeral mechanism has been suggested, since significant increases of IgM and IgG antibodies have been found in patients with disc prolapse.[4, 33] As yet, no immunoglobulins have been found in the disc tissue removed at the time of surgery.

The fact that the interaction of mechanical and inflammatory components yields signs and symptoms of the various lumbar disc syndromes is inescapable; however, specifics concerning the dynamics of that interaction remain hypothetical at this time.

Leg Pain

The patient notes a sharp, lancinating pain, usually starting in the proximal portion of the leg and ultimately progressing distally in a pattern typical of a dermatome. The L5 and S1 spinal nerves are most frequently involved, reflecting the fact that the greatest number of disc herniations occur at L4–L5 and L5–S1, respectively.[35, 39] The onset of leg pain may be insidious or extremely dramatic and associated with a tearing or snapping sensation in the spine; however, the insidious presentation is more typical for both the first sciatic attacks and those that precipitated the surgical intervention.[43]

At the onset of the sciatica, back pain may suddenly abate. The mechanical explanation of this is that once the annulus has ruptured, it is no longer placed under tension, and there is no longer a stimulus for pain in the lower back.

When the sciatic pain is acute, the patient or patient's family may note that he is listing, usually away from the side of the sciatica, Occasionally, if the disc herniation is axillary or central in position, the patient may list toward the side of his sciatica. Both maneuvers obviously tend to decrease tension on the compromised nerve root.

The pain is frequently made worse by any action that increases intraspinal pressures, such as the Valsalva maneuver, coughing and sneezing, and bearing down during defecation; this clinical correlate is better understood with Nachemson's in vivo disc pressure studies.[31]

The patient may be aware of a marked limitation of motion in the spine, and he often states that his back is "locked." This is particularly true in adolescents with disc hernations.[6, 7] In extreme cases, the pain may prevent the patient from placing any stress on the back or leg, and the individual may lie helpless on the floor or in bed with the feeling that he is "paralyzed," whereas in reality the limiting factor is pain. In high disc lesions affecting the fourth lumbar spinal nerves, the pain may be isolated to the area of the knee, and the patient may protest vigorously that the difficulty is confined only to the knee joint and may discourage any examination of his lumbar spine. When the clinical course has progressed to motor weakness involving the quadriceps muscle, the patient may complain of buckling of the knee in addition to the knee pain, which makes the situation still more confusing.

Motor Symptoms

Infrequently, patients may present with weakness in the lower extremities as their outstanding symptom; the weakness is disabling yet without pain or clinically appreciated sphincter disturbances. This is particularly true with lesions affecting the fourth and fifth anterior roots.

If the fifth nerve is compromised, the patient may note weakness on dorsiflexion of the foot and toes and occasionally have a "complete footdrop." It should be noted that in patients with a "footdrop" from an L5 root lesion, there is sparing of the tibialis anterior, which has an L4 root supply. This is in contrast to the footdrop secondary to peroneal nerve paralysis in which the tibialis anterior is also weak. Furthermore, in the L5 root syndrome, the hip abductors may be similarly affected, yielding an abductor lurch with an associated positive Trendelenburg sign. Hakelius and Hindmarsh[18] found an equal number of disc hernations in patients with isolated dorsiflexion weakness compared with patients who also had other neurologic signs. Nonetheless, a relatively painless monoradicular or, particularly, multiradicular paresis must include a differential diagnosis of a metabolic or infectious neuropathy or space-occupying lesion of the cord itself.

Disc Syndromes

SCIATIC PAIN

It is not uncommon with the acute extrusion of a fragment of nuclear material against a nerve root to have the sudden onset of sciatica without concomitant back pain. The diagnosis of discogenic disease is suggested when leg pain is aggravated by the Valsalva maneuver — a clinical correlate of increased intradiscal pressure and neural irritation. This, of course, would not be present in leg pain caused by disorders of the joints of the lower extremities or lesions of the sciatic nerve itself. Although the patient may be free of back pain, he may have marked list, muscle spasm, and limitation of motion in the lumbar spine. This is particularly true of extreme lateral lumbar disc herniations.[2] The limited lumbar mobility is not purely a defensive and learned reaction to discogenic and radicular pain but may be a manifestation of intrinsic neuromuscular pathology. Fidler and coworkers[15] found that when biopsy specimens of the multifidus muscles from patients with positive root signs were subjected to histologic

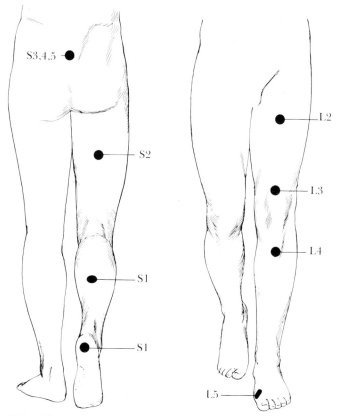

Figure 3–5. Pain may radiate to small, isolated, specific areas along the course of a dermatome. (From Rothman, R. H., and Simeone, F. A.: The Spine, 2nd ed. Philadelphia, W. B. Saunders Co., 1982.)

studies designed to differentiate slow fibers (low levels of myosin ATPase activity), which function primarily in a postural role, from fast fibers, which function more dynamically, there was a higher ratio of slow to fast fibers than is normally found. The cross-sectional area of the fast fibers was also increased. These findings, which are different from the pattern usually found in normal individuals and with aging, were interpreted as reflecting a selective injury to fast fiber motor neurons as a result of either ischemia or mechanical injury at the anterior root of the involved spinal nerve.

It should be pointed out that some patients note isolated areas of pain in the lower extremities rather than the typical pattern of dermatome involvement. The primary complaint of these individuals may be pain of the knee, calf, ankle, or heel (Fig. 3–5). In studying pain and spinal root lesions, Friis and colleagues[16] have found that approximately 10 per cent of patients with L5 or S1 lesions in particular had asymptomatic areas of dermatome between painful foci. The unwary examiner who fails to perform a meticulously thorough examination with the patient completely undressed can obviously be led astray in these instances.

Most sciatic syndromes secondary to acute disc herniations begin with pain in a proximal portion of the leg (i.e., the buttock or posterior thigh) and progress distally to involve the leg and foot. When the progression of symptoms is reversed (i.e., beginning in the foot and progressing centrally), the physician must consider the possibility of thoracic cord involvement. Sciatic pain caused by disc hernia is classically heightened by maneuvers that flex the lumbar spine and hip, such as sitting. This is in contrast with the sciatic pain resulting from spinal stenosis, which is intensified by extension of the spine. Aggravation of the pain with walking (neurogenic claudication) is more characteristic of spinal stenosis, but this is not absolutely so, and it is occasionally seen in acute disc hernations.

BACK PAIN ALONE

It has been pointed out that most patients with discogenic pain have intermittent episodes of back pain at the onset of their clinical course. Many of these individuals may proceed through the entire natural history of their disease and never experience sciatica. During acute exacerbation, pain will be accentuated by the Valsalva maneuver, and the patient will have the typical findings in the lumbar area that are noted with degenerative disc disease. In this group of patients, great judgment must be exercised before surgical intervention is elected. It is far too easy to place patients with lumbar pain into this category without careful diagnostic evaluation. The treating physician must discipline himself to rule out other causes of back pain, such as tumor, infection, and intra-abdominal disease, before this diagnostic category is used.

With the passage of time, the character of the pain changes and the acute intermittent episodes of back pain are gradually replaced by a sensation of stiffness and discomfort that is more constant but less disabling to the patient.

NEUROGENIC CLAUDICATION

With increased awareness of this syndrome, which was first appreciated by Verbiest[41] in 1954, many more patients are benefiting from a correct diagnosis of the cause of their leg pain. Vague leg pain, dysesthesias, and paresthesias distributed over the anterior and posterior thighs and calves are classically induced by spinal postures that mechanically compromise the neural canal and the neural foramina. Less often, this syndrome is precipitated by the increased metabolic and vascular demands of the lower extremities with walking and is caused by compromise of neural blood flow,[13, 45] although a combined mechanism is feasible.

Ischemia to the cauda equina is most probably the final pathway of the syndrome, but it is the postural type of neurogenic claudication that has been best defined. It must be differentiated from the claudication resulting from muscle ischemia secondary to aortofemoral disease.

The clinical presentation of neurogenic claudication is well documented.[12, 46] Patients of either sex, usually not before the fifth decade of life, will first appreciate vague pains, dysesthesia, and paresthesias with ambulation and will find excellent relief of their symptoms with a sitting or supine posture. The increased lordotic stance that is assumed with walking, particularly while walking down grades, is most likely causative. This

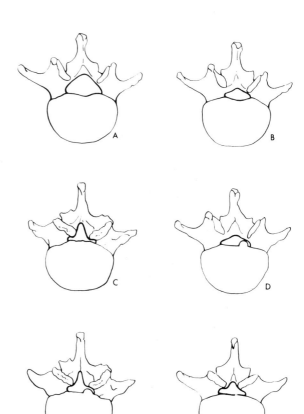

Figure 3–6. Types of lumbar spinal stenosis. *A*, Normal canal; *B*, Congenital/developmental stenosis; *C*, Degenerative stenosis; *D*, Congenital/developmental stenosis with disc herniation; *E*, Degenerative stenosis with disc herniation; *F*, Congenital/developmental stenosis with superimposed degenerative stenosis. (From Arnoldi, C. C., et al.: Lumbar spinal stenosis and nerve root entrapment syndromes. Clin. Orthop. *115*:4, 1976.)

TABLE 3–1. **Differences Between Spinal Stenosis and Disc Hernia**

Onset	Disc Hernia	Spinal Stenosis
Pain pattern	Acute ↑ with sitting ↑ with flexion	Insidious ↑ with walking ↑ with extension
Response to conservative treatment	Often	Poor
Age	30 to 50	> 60
X-ray	Normal	Spinal stenosis
Myelography	Asymmetric defect	Symmetric defect

symptomatic relationship to posture has been verified with the "bicycle test" of Van Gelderan,[9] in which claudication symptoms are not produced while the patient is on the bicycle, since there is a reduction of the lumbar lordosis and a subsequent increase in the central sagittal and foraminal dimensions of the canal. In contrast, vascular claudication symptoms will be produced with ambulation on an upgrade, which increases metabolic demands and is not avoided by stress on the bicycle. The absence of pulses below the hips and rubor and pallor changes with elevation are classic for vascular and not neurogenic claudication. In cases in which the diagnosis is uncertain, arteriography may be indicated. Provocation of a neurologic deficit with brisk walking is also helpful in the differential diagnosis, indicating a neurogenic origin.

With the maturation of the syndrome, symptoms will occur at rest, and muscle weakness, atrophy, and asymmetric reflex changes may be appreciated; however, as long as the symptoms are only aggravated dynamically, abnormal neurologic findings may be found only after stressing the patient.

The clinical syndrome has been associated with lumbar spine stenosis and nerve root entrapment syndromes. An internationally accepted classification of the anatomic syndrome (Fig. 3–6) has been defined, and the production of symptoms has been attributed to those changes occurring locally, segmentally, or generally in the affected osseous and soft tissue. However, it is important to realize that structural changes in the spinal and foraminal canals that are exaggerated with posture are, as noted by Verbiest, "conditions, but not absolute determinants of intermittent claudication."[42] Indeed, the symptoms manifested may vary significantly in individuals with similar pathomorphologic changes owing to the temporal framework within which the neural compression has occurred, the individual susceptibility of the nerves involved, and the unique functional demands and pain tolerance of the patient.

THE CAUDA EQUINA SYNDROME

Occasionally a large midline disc herniation may compress several roots of the cauda equina. Raaf[35] reported an incidence of 2 per cent of 624 patients with protruded discs; Spangfort[39] reported 1.2 per cent of 2500 cases and his review of the literature found a total incidence of approximately 2.4 per cent. He also determined no noticeable differences in sex distribution or age and found L4 and L5 discs to be the most common offending herniations but with a significantly higher number of high lumbar herniations than were found in other disc syndromes. Peyser and Harari[34] reviewed the literature and found an extremely high (11 out of 17 cases) occurrence of cauda equina syndrome when there was an intradural rupture of the intervertebral disc. These herniations occur predominantly in the high lumbar areas and, fortunately, have a very low incidence of approximately 0.2 per cent of all disc herniations.

If the lesion reaches a large size, it may mimic an intraspinal tumor, particularly if it has been slowly progressing. Often, back or perianal pain will predominate, and radicular symptoms may be masked. Difficulty with urination, consisting of frequency or overflow incontinence, may develop relatively early. In males, a history of recent impotence may be elicited by the probing examiner. If leg pain develops, it may be followed by numbness of the feet and difficulty in walking. The large midline disc

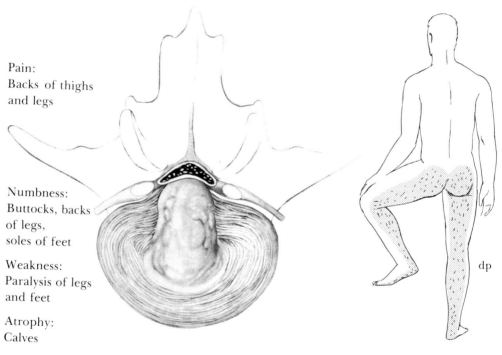

Pain:
Backs of thighs
and legs

Numbness:
Buttocks, backs
of legs,
soles of feet

Weakness:
Paralysis of legs
and feet

Atrophy:
Calves

Paralysis:
Bladder and bowel

dp

Figure 3–7. Massive herniation at the level of the third, fourth or fifth disc may cause severe compression of the cauda equina. Pain is confined chiefly to the buttocks and the back of the thighs and legs. Numbness is widespread from the buttocks to the soles of the feet. Motor weakness or loss is present in the legs and feet with loss of muscle mass in the calves. The bladder and bowels are paralyzed. (From DePalma, A. F., and Rothman, R. H.: The Intervertebral Disc. Philadelphia, W. B. Saunders Co., 1970.)

lesions, which ordinarily produce a complete myelographic block when associated with these symptoms, compress several spinal nerve roots. When compromised, the centrally placed sacral fibers to the lower abdominal viscera produce symptoms that characterize cauda equina compression. Perianal numbness and loss of the anal or bulbocavernosus reflex characterize an advanced cauda equina syndrome. Sensory deficit is typical and is frequently situated higher than the motor level.

Confusion as to the exact definition of the lesion will be encountered because the lesion will frequently be incomplete in evolving. It has been reported presenting infrequently as a lower motor neuron lesion or more frequently with abnormal radicular signs with normal or upper motor neuron lesion activity.[28] The latter lesion can be explained only on a vascular basis, but the specific mechanism in the cases reported was purely speculative.

This entity is significant in that it must be considered a reason for prompt surgical intervention, since spontaneous neurologic recovery has not been observed. If incontinence is present, only surgery, undertaken promptly, can offer a chance to lessen the hazards of possible future urinary drainage problems. Similarly, sudden severe paresis or paraplegia merits immediate and generous decompression. When the symptoms are florid, a careful preoperative myelogram for level identification with insertion of only a small amount of contrast medium is indicated, since a complete block can be anticipated (Fig. 3–7).

BLADDER SYMPTOMS

It has been recently recognized that disc protrusions may present as an abnormality of bowel and bladder function in patients with minimal or absent back pain and sciatica. It has been well documented by Emmet and Love[11] and by Ross and Jameson[37] that disc disease should be ruled out in young or middle-aged patients who develop problems of urinary retention, vesical irritability, or incontinence. This is particularly true in the absence of infection or other pelvic abnormalities.

Four syndromes have been described in regard to bladder abnormalities caused by disc derangement. They are (1) total urinary retention, (2) chronic long-standing partial retention, (3) vesicular irritability, and (4) loss of desire to void associated with an unawareness of the necessity to void. Jones and Moore[20] felt that the uninhibited type of neuropathic bladder dysfunction without loss of bladder sensation represents the incipient stage of an evolving bladder disorder caused by increasing involvement of the sacral roots.

Sharr, Garfield, and Jenkins[38] have recently emphasized the occurrence of bladder dysfunction with spinal stenosis, particularly of the degenerative variety. Although the same neuropathic bladders were encountered as in the disc herniation group, intermittency of symptoms was emphasized, therefore adding another feature to the weakness, dysesthesia, and paresthesias already associated with intermittent neurogenic claudication.

If these symptoms, particularly in their more subtle forms, are not specifically sought, they will often be overlooked.

Cystoscopy and cystometrogram, in conjunction with the myelogram, are most helpful in obtaining a definite diagnosis. These clinical syndromes are unlikely to occur with monoradicular involvement.

PHYSICAL EXAMINATION

Inspection

Limitation of motion is usually noted during the symptomatic phase of lumbar disc disease. The range of motion should be noted not only in forward and lateral flexion and extension but also in rotation. The examiner must not equate flexion of the hips with flexion of the lumbar

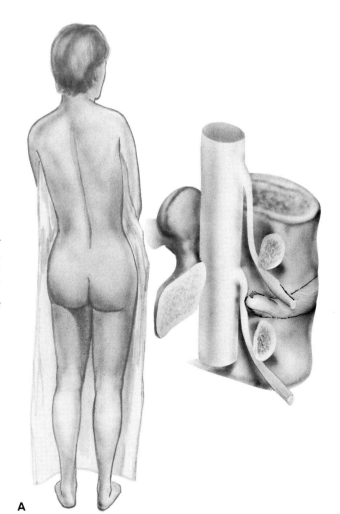

Figure 3–8. *A,* Herniation of the disc lateral to the nerve root. This will usually produce a sciatic list away from the side of the irritated nerve root.
Illustration continued on following page

A

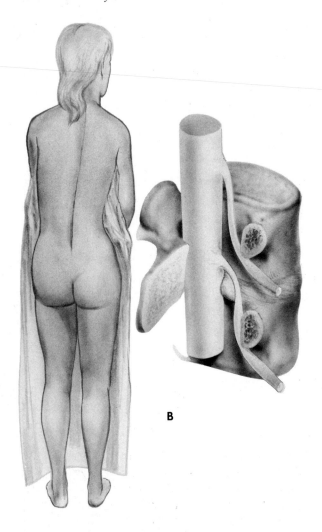

Figure 3–8. *Continued*
B, Herniation of the disc medial to the nerve root and in an axillary position. This will usually produce a sciatic list toward the side of the irritated nerve root. (From Rothman, R. H., and Simeone, F. A.: The Spine, 2nd ed. Philadelphia, W. B. Saunders Co., 1982.)

B

spine, and attention should be directed to whether reversal of the normal lumbar lordosis occurs. It has been previously noted that even in patients who have only sciatica, marked restriction of motion may be present in the lumbar spine.

When acute sciatica is present, the patient usually lists away from the side of the sciatica, producing a "sciatic scoliosis" (Fig. 3–8). When the disc herniation is lateral to the nerve root, the patient will incline away from the side of the irritated nerve in an attempt to draw the nerve root away from the disc fragment. This is dramatically demonstrated in patients with extreme lateral disc herniations in that efforts at lateral bending to the side of the lesion will markedly exaggerate the patient's pain and paresthesias.[47, 59]

In a contrary fashion, when the herniation is in an axillary position medial to the nerve root, the patient will list toward the side of the lesion, also in an effort to decompress the nerve root. This guideline to the location of disc protrusion is not absolute.

The gait and stance of patients with acute disc syndrome are also characteristic. The patient usually holds the painful leg in a flexed position and is reluctant to place his foot directly on the floor. Presumably, flexion of the leg relaxes the sciatic nerve roots and is an involuntary effort at decompression of the root. When walking, the patient has an antalgic gait, putting as little weight as possible on the extremity and quickly transferring his weight to the unaffected side. Gait disturbances as well as significant loss of lumbar motility are very characteristic of disc herniation, particularly in adolescents.[2]

Loss of normal lumbar lordosis and paravertebral muscle spasm are also usually seen during the acute phase of the disease. These abnormalities are readily appreciated on inspection, particularly the contracted and spastic mass of paravertebral muscles seen in extreme cases. Occasionally, in less acute situations, the muscle spasm can be elicited only when the patient is stressed by prolonged standing or forward flexion of the spine. Muscle spasm may on occasion be appreciated only unilaterally, and frequently this is strongly indicative of extreme lateral disc protrusion.[59]

Palpation and Percussion

Palpation of the lumbar spine in the midline usually elicits pain at the level of the symptomatic degenerative disc. It is not unusual to find tenderness laterally along the iliac crest and the iliolumbar ligament and over the sacroiliac joint. In many instances, this tenderness does not reflect disease in these lateral areas but rather hyperesthesia from nerve root irritation. Occasionally, no tenderness is elicited with palpation of the lumbar spine in the erect position, and it is necessary to have the patient flex his spine to apply pressure in the midline and then to direct him to extend his spine. This may produce marked pain in certain instances.

When spasm is present, palpation will reveal significant hardness in the contracted muscle mass. This area will frequently be exquisitely tender on firm palpation. In less marked cases of paravertebral muscle spasm, palpation should not be directed over the muscle belly but should start in the midline, with pressure exerted laterally in order to appreciate the subtle differences in muscle tone.

Palpation over the facet joints 1 to 3 cm. from the midline will frequently elicit tenderness, particularly in patients who have symptomatic degenerative joint disease with or without symptoms of spinal stenosis. This tenderness is exaggerated on palpation with extension of the spine, which increases the lumbar lordosis.

Percussion of the lumbar spine either may elicit local pain or, more significantly, may reproduce sciatica when nerve root compression is present. As with many of the previously noted findings, it is suggestive but not pathognomonic of a herniated disc.

Palpation should also be performed in the sciatic notch, along the course of the sciatic nerve itself. Hyperesthesia along the nerve is often found, and in addition, local tumors of the nerve may be discovered in this manner.

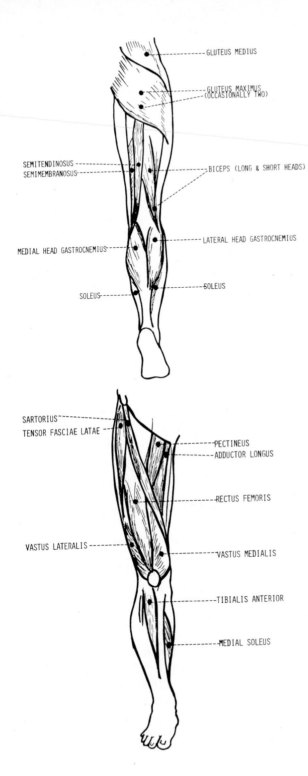

GLUTEUS MEDIUS

GLUTEUS MAXIMUS
(OCCASIONALLY TWO)

SEMITENDINOSUS
SEMIMEMBRANOSUS

BICEPS (LONG & SHORT HEADS)

MEDIAL HEAD GASTROCNEMIUS

LATERAL HEAD GASTROCNEMIUS

SOLEUS

SOLEUS

SARTORIUS
TENSOR FASCIAE LATAE

PECTINEUS
ADDUCTOR LONGUS

RECTUS FEMORIS

VASTUS LATERALIS

VASTUS MEDIALIS

TIBIALIS ANTERIOR

MEDIAL SOLEUS

Figure 3–9. Motor points of the lower extremities. (From Gunn, C. C., Chir, B., and Milbrant, W. E.: Tenderness at motor points: A diagnostic and prognostic aid for low-back injury. J. Bone Joint Surg. (Am.) *58*:815, 1976.)

The presence of tender motor points (Fig. 3–9) in the lower extremities is probably of diagnostic and prognostic importance. These represent the main neural muscular junction in the involved muscle groups, and they are reliably constant from one patient to another in their anatomic position. Diagnostically, Gunn and others[52] have found that all patients with signs and symptoms of a radiculopathy had tender motor points in the myotome corresponding to the probable segmental level of nerve root involvement.

Prognostically, in the absence of radicular signs, patients with back pain who have tender motor points remain disabled nearly three times as long as those patients without tenderness. If a radiculopathy is present with the back pain, the disability is nearly four times as long. Frequently, this tenderness has been misinterpreted as a thrombophlebitis, particularly when it is in the calf.

Neurologic Examination

A meticulous neurologic examination will yield objective evidence of nerve root compression. It will suggest the level of disc herniation but is not conclusive in this regard. The two most common levels of disc herniation are L4–L5 and L5–S1. The L3–L4 disc level is the next most common. Disc herniations at L5–S1 will usually compromise the first sacral nerve root. Similarly, a disc herniation at L4–L5 will most often compress the fifth lumbar root, whereas herniation at L3–L4 will more frequently involve the fourth lumbar root (Table 3–2). However, owing to variation in the root configuration and the position of the herniation itself, disc herniation, particularly at L4–L5, can affect not only the fifth lumbar nerve but may involve the first sacral nerve as well. In extreme lateral herniations, the nerve exiting at the same level as the disc will be involved; that is, with an L4 disc herniation, the L4 nerve root would be compressed on its course out of the neural foramina at that level. The pattern of neurologic involvement will frequently be more confusing when, in addition to a disc herniation, there is superimposed facet arthritis with lateral encroachment of the foramina. For example, with the most typical pattern of spinal

TABLE 3–2. Nerve Root Patterns*

L4 Nerve Root
1. *Pain and numbness* — L4 dermatome, posterolateral aspect of thigh, across patella, anteromedial aspect of leg
2. *Weakness and atrophy* — weak extension of knee and quadriceps muscle atrophy
3. *Reflex* — depression of patellar reflex

L5 Nerve Root
1. *Pain and numbness* — L5 dermatome, posterior aspect of thigh, anterolateral aspect of leg, medial aspect of foot and great toe
2. *Weakness and atrophy* — weak dorsiflexion of foot and toes and atrophy of anterior compartment of leg
3. *Reflex* — none, or absent posterior tibial tendon reflex

S1 Nerve Root
1. *Pain and numbness* — S1 dermatome, posterior aspect of thigh, posterior aspect of leg, posterolateral aspect of foot, lateral toes
2. *Weakness and atrophy* — weak plantar flexion of foot and toes and atrophy of posterior compartment of leg
3. *Reflex* — depression of Achilles reflex

---

*From Rothman, R. H., and Simeone, F. A.: The Spine, 2nd ed. Philadelphia, W. B. Saunders Co., 1982.

stenosis at the L4–L5 level, there may be compression of the L4 nerve root far laterally in the foramina between the arthritic facet joint, the bulging annulus, and the minor subluxation of the bodies of L4 and L5 that is frequently seen. Somewhat more medially, the L5 root may be compromised at this level by the arthritic and subluxed facet joints in the area of the lateral recess. It is more important to appreciate the spatial relations in the foramina and lateral recesses when planning one's exploration for decompression of the L4 and L5 roots in spinal stenosis.

For this reason, the authors believe that when surgery is indicated, myelography should be performed to further localize the level of lesion even though the neurologic picture is well defined. If myelography cannot be performed, exploration of at least L4–L5 and L5–S1 is mandatory. This is particularly important in view of the fact that there may be a disc herniation at more than one level, although this would be most unusual.

Motor Findings

Compression of the motor fibers of the nerve root results in weakness or paralysis of the muscle group associated with loss of tone and loss of mass of the muscle belly. Usually, a group of muscles rather than a particular muscle is involved. The patient may not be aware of this weakness until the loss is rather profound. With compression of the first sacral nerve root, little motor involvement is noted other than an occasional weakness in flexion of the foot and great toe. With compromise of the fifth lumbar nerve root, weakness primarily of the great toe and other toe extensors and less often of the evertors and dorsiflexors of the foot is noted, with atrophy of the anterior and lateral compartment of the leg. With compression of the fifth lumbar nerve root, the quadriceps muscle is frequently affected, and the patient may note weakness of extension of the knee and, more often, instability of the knee. Atrophy is usually prominent.

One must keep in mind that motor weakness may be a manifestation of a metabolic peripheral neuropathy such as diabetes. Clinically, the differentiation can be made since the paresis associated with compromise of the fifth spinal nerve will frequently spare the tibialis anterior, whereas in a diabetic peroneal neuropathy, the muscle will usually be involved. Furthermore, the presence of a Trendelenburg sign due to gluteus medius denervation resulting from a fifth lumbar radiculopathy would not be present with a diabetic peroneal neuropathy. Electromyogram (EMG) is also helpful in solving the problem of differentiating a diabetic peroneal neuropathy from the L5 root syndrome. A more diffuse pattern may be evident on EMG than can be detected clinically, indicating metabolic disease.

Sensory Changes

The pattern of sensory involvement when nerve root compression is present usually follows the dermatome of the affected nerve root. The sensory pattern of the thigh and buttocks is less specific than of the leg and the foot. With compression of the fourth lumbar nerve root, sensory abnormalities may be noted in the anteromedial aspect of the leg. With compromise of the fifth lumbar nerve root, sensory abnormalities would be noted in the anterior lateral portion of the leg and along the medial aspect of the foot to the great toe. Radiculopathy of S1 usually involves sensory abnormalities in the posterior aspect of the calf and lateral aspect of the foot.

Reflex Changes

The deep tendon reflexes are frequently altered in nerve root compression syndromes. The Achilles reflex is diminished or absent with compression of the first sacral nerve root, although Hakelius and Hindmarsh[53] noted that the incidence of disc herniation among patients whose Achilles reflex was absent was higher than among those in whom this reflex was simply diminished. Compression of the fifth lumbar nerve root most commonly causes no reflex change, but on occasion a diminution in the posterior tibial reflex can be detected. It is important to note, however, that the absence of this reflex must be asymmetric to have any clinical significance. Involvement of the fourth lumbar nerve root classically results in a decrease or absence of the patellar tendon reflex; however, it is quite common to find an L4-L5 disc herniation resulting in this patellar tendon abnormality.[53]

At the actual eliciting of the reflexes, it is suggested that several tendon taps be performed in order to assess the true amplitude of a response. Frequently, one may actually be able to fatigue a reflex response when the involved reflex arc is compromised from disc herniation.

The reader should again be reminded that many etiologic factors other than disc herniation can produce abnormalities of the deep tendon reflexes. Indeed, on a statistical basis, absence of the Achilles reflex is more often a concomitant of advanced age than of a radiculopathy.

Straight Leg Raising Test and Its Variants

There are several maneuvers that tighten the sciatic nerve and, in doing so, further compress an inflamed nerve root against a herniated lumbar disc. An excellent comprehensive view of the so-called "tension signs" in lumbar disc prolapse has been presented by Scham and Taylor.[60] With the straight leg raising maneuver, the L5 and S1 nerve roots move 2 to 6 mm. at the level of the foramina. Whether this is a true sliding movement of the nerve or passive deformation of the nerve within the neural canal and foramina[49] is debatable. What is important, however, is that when the straight leg raising test is performed in a patient with a ventral compromise of the canal or foramen, the involved nerve is subject to a tensile or compressive force, or both, to which it cannot accommodate without producing radicular symptoms. The L4 nerve root moves a lesser

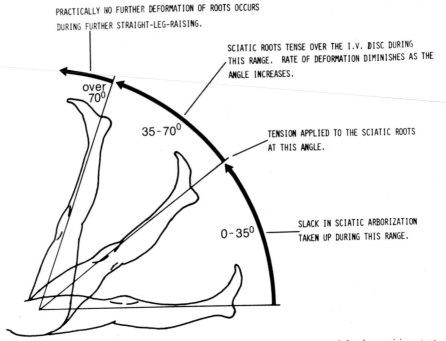

PRACTICALLY NO FURTHER DEFORMATION OF ROOTS OCCURS
DURING FURTHER STRAIGHT-LEG-RAISING.

SCIATIC ROOTS TENSE OVER THE I.V. DISC DURING
THIS RANGE. RATE OF DEFORMATION DIMINISHES AS THE
ANGLE INCREASES.

over 70°

35-70°

TENSION APPLIED TO THE SCIATIC ROOTS
AT THIS ANGLE.

0-35°

SLACK IN SCIATIC ARBORIZATION
TAKEN UP DURING THIS RANGE.

Figure 3–10. This figure illustrates the dynamics of the straight leg raising test. (Modified from Fahrni, W. H.: Observations on straight leg raising, with special reference to nerve root adhesions. Can. J. Surg. *9*:44, 1966.)

distance, and the more proximal roots show little motion. Thus, the straight leg raising test is of most importance and value in lesions of the fifth lumbar and first sacral nerve roots.

Fahrni[51] has analyzed the dynamics of the straight leg raising test and has noted that tension is realized within the nerve roots contributing to the sciatic nerve at 35 to 70 degrees of elevation from the supine position. Since deformation after 70 degrees of elevation occurs in the sciatic nerve distal to the neural foramina, any radicular pain precipitated at this elevation should not be attributed to the sequela of degenerative disc disease (Fig. 3–10).

In a review of 2000 patients with operatively proved disc herniations, the straight leg raising sign was positive in 90 per cent. Younger patients were shown to have a marked propensity for a positive straight leg raising test, although the test itself is not pathognomonic.[61] However, a negative test most probably excludes the presence of a herniated disc. After the age of 30, the negative straight leg raising test no longer excludes this diagnosis (Fig. 3–11).

The straight leg raising test is performed with the patient supine and the head flat or on a low pillow. The examiner's hand is placed on the ilium to stabilize the pelvis, and the other hand slowly elevates the leg by the heel with the knee straight. The patient should be questioned as to whether this produces leg pain. Only when leg pain or radicular symptoms are produced is this test considered positive. Back pain alone is not a positive finding in this maneuver.

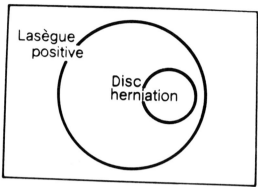

Age: under 30 years

Figure 3–11. These Venn diagrams illustrate the marked propensity for a positive Lasègue test with disc herniation in the young. Over the age of 30 the propensity decreases, although the specificity increases for this test in disc herniation. (From Spangfort, E.: Lasègue's sign in patients with lumbar disc herniation. Acta Orthop., *42*:459, 1971.)

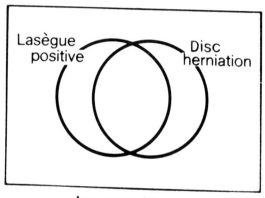

Age: over 30 years

Many variations of this test have been described. The knee may first be flexed to 90 degrees and the hip then flexed to 90 degrees. Next, the knee is gradually extended. If this maneuver produces leg pain, the test is considered positive. Both this test and the straight leg raising test have been attributed to Lasègue. Fajersztajn[60] described a variation to the straight leg raising test in which the foot is dorsiflexed. This not only may produce an exacerbation of the pain produced in the straight leg raising test but also could reproduce radicular pain when the conventional straight leg raising test was negative.

MacNab[56] feels that the most reliable test of root tension is the bowstring sign, which is another manifestation of the straight leg raising test. The straight leg raising test is performed as usual until pain is elicited. At this point, however, the knee is flexed, which will usually significantly reduce symptoms. Finger pressure is applied to the popliteal space over the terminal aspect of the sciatic nerve, and this will re-establish the painful radicular symptoms.

The sitting root test is yet another variation on this theme. With the patient sitting and the cervical spine flexed, the knee is extended while the hip remains flexed to 90 degrees. The patient may complain of leg pain or may attempt to extend his hip, again indicating nerve root tension.

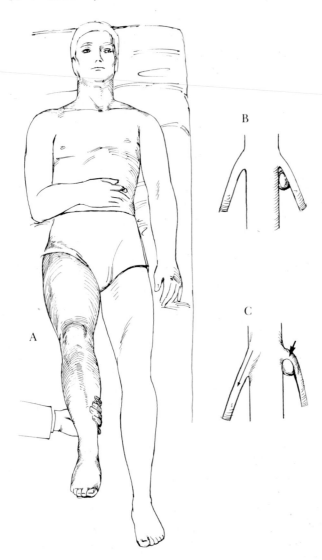

Figure 3–12. Movement of nerve roots when the leg on the opposite side is raised. *A,* When the leg is raised on the unaffected side the roots on the opposite side slide slightly downward and toward the midline. *B* and *C,* In the presence of a disc lesion, this movement increases the root tension. (From De-Palma, A. F., and Rothman, R. H.: The Intervertebral Disc. Philadelphia, W. B. Saunders Co., 1970.)

Medial rotation of the hip joint can also apply tension to the sacral plexus in the supine posture. Troup and Breig[62] reported that sciatic pain could be reproduced when medial hip rotation was performed at the pain-free limits of the straight leg raising test.

The contralateral straight leg raising test is performed in the same manner as the straight leg raising test, except that the nonpainful leg is raised. If this produces sciatica in the opposite extremity, the test is considered positive. This is very suggestive of a herniated disc and also is an indication of the location of the extrusion. Hudgins[54] reported that this sign was positive in 97 per cent of patients with surgically confirmed disc herniations. The prolapse will often be large but not in the usual lateral position. At surgery, the disc will usually be found medial to the nerve root in the axilla (Fig. 3–12).

It should be noted that when the roots of the femoral nerve are involved, they are tensed not by the straight leg raising test but by the reverse straight leg raising test, that is, by hip extension and knee flexion. This is usually performed while the patient is prone or positioned laterally with the unaffected side down. As with the straight leg raising test, there is a contralateral femoral traction sign.[50]

Peripheral Vascular Examination

No examination of a patient with back or leg pain can be considered complete without evaluation of the peripheral circulation. There should be an examination of the posterior tibial and dorsalis pedis arteries, as well as a determination of the skin temperature and an inspection for the presence of the atrophic changes seen with ischemic disease.

In addition to the peripheral vascular examination, several other clinical findings as well as the patient's history will usually help differentiate vascular claudication from intermittent neurogenic claudication. In the unusual case in which the patient's history and physical findings could be compatible with both types of claudication, quantitative studies of the arterial system and consultation with a vascular surgeon would be indicated.

Hip Joint Examination

The clinician can usually differentiate intra-articular hip disease from symptomatic degenerative disc disease. Limitation of range of motion of the hip, particularly in rotation, along with groin discomfort, is most indicative of hip disease. Furthermore, during examination of the hip, coincident hip flexion and knee extension should not elicit any tension signs implicating nerve root tension. If the patient's symptom complex in the thigh and leg are reproduced with rotation of the hip, this would certainly indicate hip pathology rather than nerve root compression as the causative factor.

It is of interest, however, that Magora[57] did find evidence of degenerative hip disease in 10 per cent of approximately 400 patients suffering from low back pain.

The piriformis muscle used in external hip rotation has been implicated as a positive cause of sciatic-like symptoms.[55, 58] This muscle runs in proximity to the sciatic nerve, and any injury to the muscle, particularly if it is anomalously bifurcated and surrounding the sciatic nerve, could precipitate local pain over the sciatic notch, as well as irritation along the course of the nerve. Tenderness over the piriformis muscle on rectal or vaginal examination, along with local and referred pain with weakness when the hip is abducted and externally rotated against resistance, is most suggestive of this syndrome. Bimanual injection of the muscle has yielded very satisfactory results.

Abdominal and Rectal Examination

Many intra-abdominal and retroperitoneal abnormalities can result in back and leg pain. Careful palpation of the abdomen together with rectal and pelvic examinations will disclose many of these lesions and lead to a correct diagnosis.

REFERENCES

CLINICAL SYNDROMES

1. Arnoldi, C. C., Brodsky, J., Cauchoix, H. V., et al.: Lumbar spinal stenosis and nerve root entrapment syndromes. Clin. Orthop., *115*:4, 1976.
2. Abdullah, A. F., Ditto, E. W., Byrd, E. B., and Williams, R.: Extreme-lateral lumbar disc herniations. J. Neurosurg., *41*:229, 1974.
3. Bernini, P. M., Rothman, R. H., and Simeone, F.: Sympathetic dystrophy complicating lumbar disc herniations. In Press. 1981.
4. Bisla, R. S., Marchisello, P. J., Lockshin, M. D., et al.: Auto-immunological basis of disk degeneration. Clin. Orthop., *121*:205, 1976.
5. Bobechko, W. T., and Hirsh, C.: Auto-immune response to nucleus pulposus in the rabbit. J. Bone Joint Surg., *47B*:574, 1965.
6. Bulos, S.: Herniated intervertebral lumbar disc in the teenager. J Bone Joint Surg., *55*:273, 1973.
7. Bradford, D. S., and Garcia, A.: Lumbar intervertebral disk herniations in children and adolescents. Orthop. Clin. North Am., *2*:583, 1971.
8. Brown, M. D., and Tsaltas, T. T.: Studies on the permeability of the intervertebral disc during skeletal maturation. Spine, *4*:240, 1976.
9. Dyck, P., and Doyle, J. B.: "Bicycle test" of van Gelderen in diagnosis of intermittent cauda equina compression syndrome. J. Neurosurg., *46*:667, 1977.
10. Elliott, F. A., and Schutta, H. S.: The differential diagnosis of sciatica. Orthop. Clin. North Am., *2*:477, 1971.
11. Emmett, J., and Love, J.: Vesical dysfunction caused by protruded lumbar disc. J. Urol., *105*:80, 1971.
12. Epstein, B. S., Epstein, J. A., and Jones, M. D.: Lumbar spinal stenosis. Radiologic Clin. North Am., *2*:227, 1977.
13. Evans, J. G.: Neurogenic intermittent claudication. Br. Med. J., *5415*:985, 1964.
14. Farfan, H. S.: Mechanical Disorders of the Low Back. Philadelphia, Lea and Febiger, 1973.
15. Fidler, M. W., Jowett, R. L., and Troup, J. D. G.: Myosin ATPase activity in multifidus muscle from cases of lumbar spinal derangement. J. Bone Joint Surg., *57*(2):220, 1975.
16. Friis, M. L., Gulliksen, G. C., Rasmussen, P., and Husby, J.: Pain and spinal root compression. Acta Neurochir., *39*:241, 1977.
17. Gertzbein, S. D., Tait, J. H., and Devlin, S. R.: The stimulation of lymphocytes by nucleus pulposus in patients with degenerative disk disease of the lumbar spine. Clin. Orthop., *123*:149, 1977.
18. Hakelius, A., and Hindmarsh, J.: The significance of neurological signs and myelographic findings in the diagnosis of lumbar root compression. Acta Orthop. Scand., *43*:239, 1972.
19. Jayson, M. I., Herbert, C. M., and Barks, J. S.: Intervertebral discs: nuclear morphology and bursting pressures. Ann. Rheum. Dis., *32*:208, 1973.
20. Jones, D. L., and Moore, T.: The types of neuropathic bladder dysfunction associated with prolapsed lumbar intevertebral discs. Br. J. Urol., *45*:39, 1973.
21. Keller, R. H.: Traumatic displacement of the cartilaginous vertebral rim: A sign of intervertebral disc prolapse. Radiology, *110*:21, 1974.
22. Kellgren, J. H.: The anatomical source of back pain. Rheum. Rehab., *16*:3, 1977.
23. Kulak, R. F., Schultz, A. B., and Belytschko, T. B.: Biomechanical characteristics of vertebral motion segments and intervertebral discs. Orthop. Clin. North Am. *6*(1):121–133, 1975.
24. Kulak, R. F., Belytschko, T. B., Schultz, A. B., and Galante, J.: Nonlinear behavior of the human intervertebral disc under axial load. J. Biomech., *9*:377, 1976.

25. MacNab, I. Personal correspondence.
26. Markolf, K. L., and Morris, J. M.: The structural components of the intervertebral disc. J. Bone Joint Surg., *4*:675, 1974.
27. Maroudas, A., Nachemson, A., Stockwell, R., and Urban, J.: In vitro studies of the diffusion of glucose into the intervertebral disc. *In* Nachemson, A.: Towards a better understanding of low back pain: A review of the mechanics of the lumbar disc. Rheum. Rehab., *14*:129, 1975.
28. Maury, M., Francois, N., and Skoda, A.: About the neurological sequelae of herniated intervertebral disc. Paraplegia, *11*:221, 1973.
29. Mooney, V., and Robertson, J.: The facet syndrome. Clin. Orthop., *115*:149, 1976.
30. Murphy, R. W.: Nerve roots and spinal nerves in degenerative disk disease. Clin. Orthop., *129*:46, 1977.
31. Nachemson, A.: The load on lumbar disks in different positions of the body. Acta Orthop. Scand., *36*:426, 1965.
32. Nachemson, A.: Towards a better understanding of low-back pain: A review of the mechanics of the lumbar disc. Rheum. Rehab., *14*:129, 1975.
33. Naylor, A.: Intervertebral disc prolapse and degeneration. The biochemical and biophysical approach. Spine, *2*:108, 1976.
34. Peyser, E., and Harari, A.: Intradural rupture of lumbar intervertebral disk: report of two cases with review of the literature. Surg. Neurol., *8*:95, 1977.
35. Raaf, J.: Some observations regarding 905 patients operated upon for protruded lumbar intervertebral disc. Am. J. Surg., *97*:388, 1959.
36. Resnick, D., and Niwayama, G.: Intervertebral disk herniations: cartilaginous (Schmorl's) nodes. Radiology, *126*:57, 1978.
37. Ross, J. C., and Jameson, R. M.: Vesical dysfunction due to prolapsed disc. Br. Med. J., *3*:752, 1971.
38. Sharr, M. M., Garfield, J. S., and Jenkins, J. D.: The association of bladder dysfunction with degenerative lumbar spondylosis. Br. J. Urol., *45*:616, 1973.
39. Spangfort, E. V.: The lumbar disc herniation. A computer-aided analysis of 2504 operations. Acta Orthop. Scand. (Suppl.), *142*:61, 1977.
40. Smyth, M. J., and Wright, V. J.: Sciatica and the intervertebral disc. An experimental study. J. Bone Joint Surg., *40A*:1401, 1958.
41. Verbiest, H.: Radicular syndrome from developmental narrowing of lumbar vertebral canal. J. Bone Joint Surg., *36B*:230, 1954.
42. Verbiest, H.: Pathomorphologic aspects of developmental lumbar stenosis. Orthop. Clin. North Am., *6*(1):177–196, 1975.
43. Weber, H. Lumbar disc herniations. A prospective study of prognostic factors including a controlled trial. J. Oslo City Hosp., *28*:33, 89, 1978.
44. Wiley, A. M., and Trueta, J.: The vascular anatomy of the spine and its relationship to pyogenic vertebral osteomyelitis. J. Bone Joint Surg., *41B*(4):796, 1959.
45. Wilson, C. B., Ehni, G., and Grollimus, J.: Neurogenic intermittent claudication. Clin. Neurosurg., *18*:62, 1971.
46. Wiltse, L. L., Kirkaldy-Wills, W. H., McIvor, G. W. D.: The treatment of spinal stenosis. Clin. Orthop., *115*:83, 1976.

PHYSICAL EXAMINATION

47. Abdullah, A. F., Ditto, E. W., Byrd, E. B., and Williams, R.: Extreme lateral disc herniations. J. Neurosurg., *41*:229, 1974.
48. Boulos, S.: Herniated intervertebral lumbar disc in the teenager. J. Bone Joint Surg., *55B*(2):273, 1973.
49. Breig, A., and Marions, O.: Biomechanics of the lumbosacral nerve roots. Acta Radiol., *1*:1141, 1963.
50. Dyck, P.: The femoral nerve traction test with lumbar disc protrusions. Surg. Neurol., *6*:163, 1976.
51. Fahrni, W. H.: Observations on straight leg raising with special reference to nerve root adhesions. Can. J. Surg., *9*:44, 1970.
52. Gunn, C. C., Chir, B., and Milbrand, W. E.: Tenderness at motor points: A diagnostic and prognostic aid to low back injury. J. Bone Joint Surg., *58A*:815, 1976.
53. Hakelius, A., and Hindmarsh, J.: The significance of neurological signs and myelography findings in the diagnosis of lumbar root compression. Acta Orthop. Scand., *43*:234, 1972.
54. Hudgins, W. R.: The crossed straight leg raising test. New Engl. J. Med., *297*:1127, 1977.

55. Kerkaldy-Willis, W. H., and Hill, R. J.: A more precise diagnosis for low back pain. Spine, *4*(2):102, 1979.

56. MacNab, I.: Backache. Baltimore, Williams & Wilkins, 1977.

57. Magora, A.: Investigation of the relation between low back pain and occupation. VII Neurologic and orthopaedic condition. Scand. J. Rehab. Med., 7:141, 1975.

58. Pace, J. B., and Neagle, D.: Piriformis syndrome. West. J. Med., *124*:435, 1976.

59. Patrick, B. S.: Extreme lateral ruptures of lumbar invertebral discs. Surg. Neurol., *3*:301, 1975.

60. Scham, S., and Taylor, T.: Tension signs in lumbar disc prolapse. Clin. Orthop., *44*:163, 1966.

61. Spangfort, E.: Lasègue's sign in patients with lumbar disc herniation. Acta Orthop., *42*:459, 1971.

62. Troup, J. D. G., and Breig, A.: The effect of medial hip rotation on the sacral plexus and its significance in the straight leg raising test. Proceedings 5th Annual Meeting of the International Society for the Study of the Lumbar Spine. San Francisco, 1978.

Chapter 4

CLINICAL APPROACH — ALGORITHM FOR THE VIRGIN BACK

ALGORITHM FOR TREATMENT OF LUMBAR DISC DEGENERATION

The task of the spinal surgeon in regard to the patient with low back pain is to return that patient to a normal functional existence as quickly as possible. The surgeon's ability to achieve that ideal goal is dependent not so much on technical excellence in the operating room as it is on the precision and accuracy of decision-making. In an effort to help physicians improve their decision-making capacities, the authors have developed a treatment algorithm to analyze these very difficult and complex situations.

The outlined plan is derived not only from the evaluation of therapeutic successes but also, and probably of greater significance, the evaluation of the genesis of the patients who have failed to respond to operative measures of treatment — the so-called "salvage back."[8] Relying heavily on these clinical data, a format and approach have been developed that will optimize therapeutic efforts by enabling the physician to base decision-making on well-delineated rules rather than emotion and intuition. Webster defines an algorithm as "a set of rules for solving a particular problem in a finite number of steps" (Fig. 4–1).

The algorithm can be followed in sequence. Assume that a treating physician has examined these individuals and has come to the conclusion after the initial interview and examination that the symptoms are secondary to lumbar disc degeneration. Presuming that these patients have not been previously treated, the overwhelming majority should be instructed to begin a course of conservative therapy. Only the patient with a frank cauda equina syndrome or unequivocal progressive motor weakness should be treated with the more aggressive line of myelography and possible surgery. The early stage of treatment of lumbar disc disease is a waiting game. The passage of time, the use of salicylates, and bed rest are the modalities that have proved to be the safest and most effective. We advise an initial period of this type of conservative treatment for up to six weeks. In our experience, only one or two patients per year justify following the pathway toward initial surgical intervention.

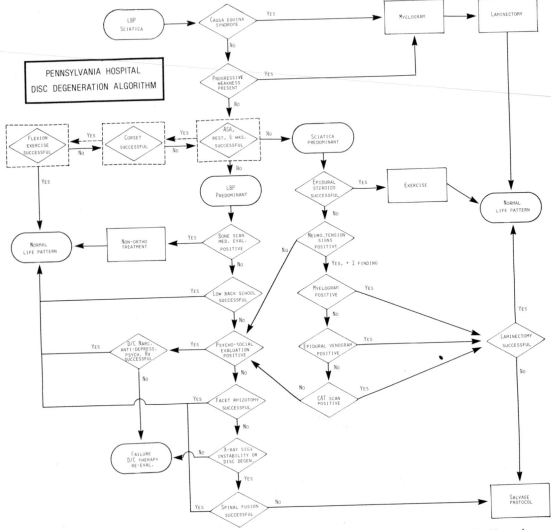

Figure 4–1. Algorithm for the treatment of lumbar disc degeneration. (From Rothman, R. H., and Simeone, F. A.: The Spine, 2nd ed. Philadelphia, W. B. Saunders Co., 1982.)

However, in the face of a frank cauda equina syndrome or truly progressive motor weakness, equivocation and procrastination are not warranted, and a vigorous recommendation for myelography is indicated. In these instances, the myelogram will almost always be clearly positive and should be promptly followed by lumbar laminectomy. One can almost always expect a dramatic resolution of pain, if not motor deficit, with prompt return to normal life patterns. Even in these patients, one might argue that the data substantiating this aggressive surgical posture are not adequate; however, at the present time, our recommendation remains as stated.

Those individuals who respond to conservative treatment after the initial encounter should be mobilized with the use of a lightweight flexible corset when they have achieved approximately 80 per cent relief of their symptoms. Once they have been able to return to increased function and are more comfortable, we would begin a program of isometric lumbar flexion exercises with subsequent return to a normal life pattern. The pathways along this portion of the algorithm are two-way streets, and should regression occur with exacerbation of symptoms, one can simply resort to more stringent conservative measures, such as returning to the use of a corset and, if necessary, further bed rest. The vast majority of patients with acute low back pain will proceed along this pathway, returning to a normal life pattern within two months from the onset of their symptoms.

Evaluation and Treatment of Sciatica and Back Pain

If the initial battery of conservative measures has failed and six weeks have passed, we would advise sorting these patients into two groups. In the first category, sciatica is predominant and in the second, low back pain predominates. In those patients in whom *low back pain* is the predominant and persisting symptom despite six weeks of conservative measures, we would advise that the patient have a technetium bone scan and complete medical evaluation by an internist. In those patients in whom *sciatica* is the predominant and persisting symptom, we would escalate our conservative therapy to include the use of epidural steroids on either an inpatient or an outpatient basis. There are many alternate types of conservative treatment available, such as traction and manipulation, but unfortunately, they have not withstood the test of scientific scrutiny and thus should not become a routine part of the treatment program.[22] There may be the occasional patient for whom traction will be utilized and even the occasional patient for whom it is helpful, but as a group, patients who are treated with traction improve no more rapidly than those who are treated simply by bed rest alone. Patients who undergo epidural steroid therapy may have one or two repeat steroid treatments. We usually allow an additional six weeks to pass before considering the epidural steroid treatment a failure.

If the epidural steroids are effective in alleviating sciatica, the patient should be started on a program of isometric lumbar flexion exercises and should be encouraged to return to a normal life pattern. Again, this pathway will usually be complete in less than three months. If the epidural steroids have not been effective and three months have passed with the patient having persistent and intolerable sciatica, surgery should be considered. At this point, one must carefully re-evaluate the patient for the presence of a neurologic deficit and a tension sign, such as the straight leg raising test or sitting root test.

DIAGNOSTIC STUDIES

It has been repeatedly documented that for surgery to be effective in the treatment of sciatica, the surgeon must find unequivocal evidence of nerve root compression at surgery. In order to predict mechanical root compression, the physician must have firm substantiation for his decision, not only in the neurologic examination but also in terms of radiographic data, before proceeding with the laminectomy.

If the patient has neither a neurologic deficit nor a positive tension sign, we feel that, regardless of the radiographic findings, there is inadequate evidence of root compression to proceed with surgery. Individuals who have unremitting complaints but a paucity of findings should be advised to have a psychosocial evaluation in an effort to explain this discrepancy.

Patients who have either a neurologic deficit or a positive tension sign are subjected to a myelogram. If the myelogram is clearly positive, surgery should be promptly undertaken. If the myelogram is negative, it is possible that a lateral disc herniation that lies beyond the dural pouch and root sleeve is present. These individuals should have an epidural venogram, which may reveal lateral herniation.[14] If the venogram is positive, surgery would be indicated and undertaken. With the increased use of water-soluble myelography, the sensitivity of myelography is much improved for L5–S1 disc herniations. Thus, the authors have recently found it far less necessary to utilize epidural venography than in the past, when oil was the contrast agent of choice. The epidural venogram still retains its usefulness in association with metrizamide myelography when the caudal sac ends above the L5–S1 level or when there are unequivocal findings on physical examination that are suggestive of disc herniation and the myelogram is normal.

If the epidural venogram is unrevealing, we would proceed to computer-assisted tomography to substantiate that there may be bony foraminal encroachment that is not seen on either the myelogram or venogram. If the scan is positive, surgery in the form of a foraminotomy would be recommended.

If all of these radiographic modalities are unrevealing, the patient would be denied surgery and proceed to a psychosocial evaluation. Exceptions to these operative criteria should be few and far between. In the authors' experience, when sympathy for the patient's complaints has outweighed objective evaluation, surgical endeavors have been fraught with great difficulty. The explorations have almost always been unrevealing and thus unrewarding. In individuals who have met these firm criteria for lumbar laminectomy, the results are overwhelmingly satisfactory, and one can expect 95 per cent of these patients to have a good or excellent result.

Patients who were originally classified as having predominantly back pain and who failed to respond to the initial program of conservative treatment will undergo a bone scan and medical evaluation by an internist. The bone scan has been found to be an excellent survey tool, often identifying early spinal tumors and infections that are not seen on routine radiographic examination. If the authors had one diagnostic study available in patient management, they would prefer the bone scan to routine radiographic examination. The internist's thorough search will frequently reveal problems such as a posterior penetrating ulcer, pancreatitis, and abdominal aneurysms that orthopedists may not have the expertise or facilities to diagnose. If these diagnostic modalities have positive results, the patient would be transferred into nonorthopedic treatment and would no longer be in our therapeutic algorithm.

LOW BACK SCHOOL

If the bone scans of these patients are not abnormal and other medical disease is not found as a cause for their back pain, they would be referred for a second level of therapy, which is the low back school. At the basis of this concept is the belief that patients with low back pain, given proper education and understanding of their disease and appropriate forms of self-administered conservative therapy, can often return to a productive and functional life. Ergonomics, the proper and efficient use of the spine in work and recreation, is stressed. This type of educational process is both inexpensive and effective, which is highly desirable.

If the low back school is effective during its four week curriculum, the patient is discharged and may return to a normal life pattern. It is critical that a patient be thoroughly screened before he is referred to this type of facility, so that the physician is not in the position of treating tumors and infections in classrooms.

PSYCHOSOCIAL EVALUATION

If the low back school is ineffective, these patients should undergo a thorough psychosocial evaluation in an attempt to explain the failure of these usually effective therapeutic measures for low back pain. The use of a psychosocial evaluation is predicted on the knowledge and belief that a patient's disability is related not only to his pathologic anatomy but also to his perception of pain and his stability in relationship to the sociologic environment. Only the most myopic physician would deny that the patient's psychologic profile and ability to function in a specific environment play a part in the treatment of low back pain. All spinal surgeons see the patient with a frank herniated disc who is able to continue working and who regards it as only a trivial and annoying problem. At the other end of the spectrum, the physician sees the hysterical patient who takes to bed immediately upon the slightest twinge of lumbago.

The type of psychosocial evaluation would depend on the needs of the patient and the facilities available to the treating physician. The type of symptoms would also dictate in part the studies required. The Minnesota Multiphasic Personality Inventory and consultation by a psychiatrist who is an expert in the treatment of chronic low back disorders are routinely utilized. In addition, the differential spinal block is administered for those persons with a significant component of leg pain, and the thiopental (Pentothal) interview is used for those whose symptoms are primarily axial in nature. At this point, it is not uncommon to discover drug habituation, depression, and other psychiatric and psychologic causes for magnification and propagation of the pain complaint. If the evaluation reveals this type of pathology, proper measures are instituted to overcome the disability. It is shocking to note the numbers of ambulatory patients who present with addiction to Percodan and Valium, alone or in combination. The authors strongly feel that the use of these drugs should be kept to an absolute minimum. Percodan is truly addicting, and Valium causes both habituation and depression. The complaint of low back pain is a common expression of depression, and to treat these individuals with Valium is not only foolish but detrimental to their welfare. In a patient whose symptoms seem to be primarily an expression of a depressive reaction, antidepressant drugs such as amitriptyline (Elavil) have been found to be very helpful. Because of the moderate side-effects that occur with the use of Elavil, the drug has been combined with the tranquilizer perphenazine (Trilafon) as Triavil. It has been the most effective antidepressant with the fewest unpleasant side-effects.

The type of psychiatric and psychologic treatment that is indicated will depend on the background of the patient, his intelligence and insight, and the means available to him to afford this type of treatment. Unfortunately, psychiatric therapy is expensive and demanding of a high level of insight and motivation. Psychologists and psychiatric clinics with ancillary personnel such as psychiatric social workers are often a reasonable answer. Programs of behavior modification such as operant conditioning have proved to be useful in certain situations in helping patients to return to a more productive way of life, but hard data supporting this therapy are not available at the present time. The patient who is unwilling or unable to follow the program that is outlined, who continues the use of narcotics, and who rejects or does not respond to the recommended psychiatric treatment must be considered a failure. Discontinuation of medical therapy would be advocated at that time. To continue random measures of treatment for these individuals without correcting their underlying psychosocial disorder is a waste of time, money, and medical facilities. They should be discharged from therapy, with the offer to re-evaluate them in one year should they wish to resume treatment. If these patients are able to give up narcotics and respond to the psychiatric counseling that is offered, they will usually be able to return to a normal life pattern without further orthopedic treatment.

Persistent Pain in Patients Without Psychosocial Abnormality

Patients who have persistent back and leg pain and in whom no psychosocial abnormality has been detected might benefit from a facet rhizotomy. This type of patient will have persistent back pain, with or without referred leg pain and without documentation of nerve root compression. Temporary relief of back pain after facet joint injection with steroids and a local anesthetic is a favorable predictive factor. This therapeutic measure has not faced the scrutiny of a double-blind prospective study, but our early investigations do show some usefulness and little potential for harm. It must be stated that the ultimate role of this modality is not yet defined and is still under study. If this treatment measure is successful, the patient can promptly return to a normal life pattern. If, on the other hand, the facet rhizotomy fails to alleviate back pain, the lumbar spine x-rays should be carefully studied for unequivocal evidence of instability or localized disc degeneration. For these purposes, instability would be defined as to-and-fro motion with flexion and extension, reversal of the normal lordotic position of the motion segment, or traction osteophytes at one level. In patients with unremitting mechanical back pain who have not responded to prolonged conservative treatment and in whom no psychosocial disorder is found, spinal fusion may be of help.

If radiographic stigmata of instability or localized disc degeneration are not present, the patient must be considered a treatment failure, and therapy should be discontinued. There are no further measures that will benefit these individuals, and they should be offered re-evaluation in one year to be certain that the clinical picture has not changed and no occult disease process has been uncovered. If the decision is made to proceed with spinal fusion, both the surgeon and the patient must be ready to accept a level of effectiveness of approximately 75 per cent. In these patients, the failure rate after spinal fusion is considerably higher than the failure rate after laminectomy for the symptoms outlined earlier. If the spinal fusion is successful, the patient should be encouraged to return quickly to a normal life pattern. If the spinal fusion has failed, the patient will proceed to the salvage protocol discussed previously. It should be emphasized that few patients will decide to have a spinal fusion, and in the authors' practices, only three to four patients per year will have an arthrodesis for disc degeneration. By far, the greater number of patients with low back pain will find improvement with conservative measures, will have nonorthopedic causes for the low back pain, or will have a psychosocial disturbance.

The authors have found that with the use of the decision-making algorithm, their patients receive the therapeutic measures that are most helpful at the optimal time and are neither denied helpful surgery nor submitted to operations that are useless surgical exercises.

CONSERVATIVE TREATMENT OF LUMBAR DISC DISEASE

The goals to be established in the nonoperative treatment of lumbar disc disease should be threefold: (1) relief of pain, (2) increase of functional capacity, and (3) slowing of the disease process.

At our present state of knowledge, the first two goals are frequently within the reach of the treating physician; the last and most important goal is not. Reports on the efficacy of various types of conservative therapy vary tremendously. One of the most optimistic of these reports claims that in a group of 400 patients with acute disc lesions, only two required operative intervention after conservative therapy.[17] Our own experience has led us to become more cautious in responding to inquiries about the possible failure of conservative therapy and the necessity for operative intervention.

Approximately 20 per cent of patients with a firm diagnosis of an acute disc hernia will ultimately require surgery when followed over a period of years. This finding is in agreement with several reports in the literature.[4, 13, 15]

The quality of result of conservative treatment of patients with disc disease will depend in part on the criteria for including a patient in this study group. Colonna and Friedenberg,[4] utilizing the strict criteria of myelographic demonstration of disc protrusion, found a relatively low recovery rate of about 30 per cent. In a similar vein, Weber's prospective study, which had strict clinical and roentgenographic prerequisites, also revealed that results at one year following conservative management were not as good as those results following surgery.[23] After four years of follow-up, however, there was no statistically significant difference between surgical and conservative management. It is of interest that the neurologic deficits that remained (excluding cauda equina syndrome and rapidly progressive deficits) after four years of follow-up were independent of the treatment modality utilized.

The question of efficacy of nonoperative treatment depends not only on the diagnostic and intellectual capabilities of the physician but also on his ability to educate the patient and render proper emotional support. Success will depend on the willingness of the patient to accept not only various levels of chronic and acute pain but also altered functional capacity. The physician must keep in mind and emphasize to the patient that disc degeneration is not a lethal disease. If the patient is willing to live with his pain, it is his prerogative to persist with the course of conservative therapy despite the treating physician's feeling that it has failed and operative intervention is required. A decision for surgical intervention should not be made ex cathedra but by the patient and his physician on the basis of mutual understanding, confidence, and trust. The patient with a bona fide neural compressive lesion who does not respond to conservative therapy in a reasonable length of time should be granted the benefit of surgical intervention to allow him to lead a more comfortable and active life.

The course of conservative therapy will be presented here as it evolved over a period of years and was found to be effective in a large patient population. The reasons for its efficacy are often hypothetical, but it has been shown on an empirical basis to be the most efficient approach to problems of acute and chronic disc lesions.

Bed Rest

The most important element of the therapy for acute lumbar disc lesions is an adequate period of bed rest. This conclusion has been derived empirically over the years and has been supported by biomechanical and clinical studies.

Nachemson has established in vivo data verifying that in the vertebral disc, pressure can be significantly reduced with the supine posture.[20] Related work by Anderson and Ortegrens[1] has demonstrated a reduction of dorsal and abdominal muscle activity as one assumes a more horizontal position. Assuming the validity of the clinical correlation of increasing pressure and increasing symptoms in the lumbar spine, bed rest would seem to be the rational first line treatment in conservative management. Disc pressures and facet joint reactive forces in the lumbar spine are a result of the summation of the force of gravity as well as associated muscle force vectors called on to provide stability in the upright stance.

Clinically, Wiesel and Rothman[25] conducted a random study on the efficacy of bed rest in acute low back in 80 basic combat trainees. All patients had back pain, but none had tension signs or neural deficits indicative of radiculopathy. While one group of 40 patients was kept at complete bed rest, the second group of 40 patients was kept ambulatory but excused from any physical activity. Both groups received acetaminophen. The bed rest group returned to full duty 50 per cent faster and experienced 60 per cent less pain than the ambulatory group.

Prescribed bed rest can be accomplished most effectively at home, where the patient is in comfortable and familiar surroundings and is cared for by his family. Should there be a lack of adequate facilities for good home care, the individual should be admitted to the hospital for this treatment. It is expected that the patient remain at complete bed rest with the exception of bathroom privileges for bowel movements once or twice a day with the use of a bedside commode or nearby toilet facility. The short period of ambulation that is necessary to reach the bathroom is frequently less stressful than the acrobatics required to use a bedpan. If a firm mattress is available, we feel that bed boards are not necessary and in many instances will actually increase the level of discomfort noted by the patient.

While in bed, the patient should be placed in a position so that his hips and knees are flexed to a moderate but comfortable degree. This has been found to be particularly necessary in disc herniations at the L4–L5 level. The patient is cautioned against sleeping in a prone position, which will result in hyperextension of the lumbar spine. A natural or synthetic "sheepskin" will provide additional comfort if the patient is to have prolonged periods of bed rest.

The duration of this period of bed rest is of prime importance. Too frequently, patients are mobilized and allowed to return to work before the inflammatory reaction of disc herniation or musculotendinous strain has subsided. When the disability is caused by an acute disc herniation, a minimum of two weeks at complete bed rest is required whether at home or in the hospital. Subsequent to this, a week to ten days of gradual mobilization is instituted if the patient has had substantial relief of pain and is free of list and paravertebral muscle spasm. It should be mentioned parenthetically that the patient with profound motor loss or with a progressive and functionally significant neurologic deficit should undergo operative intervention; he is not a candidate for conservative therapy. It is unrealistic to expect a patient with frank disc herniation to return to full activities in less than one month. Compromise on this point is frequently sought by the patient, but in the long run, it will not be to his benefit. It should be pointed out to the patient that operative intervention in itself requires a prolonged period of rehabilitation and that strict adherence to a conservative program may preclude the necessity of operative intervention.

Based on present day knowledge of the pathophysiology of disc degeneration, it is the authors' feeling that the modality of bed rest is important so that the secondary inflammatory reaction to disc degeneration may subside. Bed rest is not instituted with the expectation that an extruded fragment will return to its original place within the annulus. Once extruded into the annulus beneath the posterior longitudinal ligament, a fragment of nuclear material does not return to its origin location. In many instances, however, if the edema and hyperemia of the soft tissues and nerve roots surrounding the extruded fragment are allowed to subside, the patient will become free of his acute back pain and sciatica. This relief may or may not be permanent. As noted earlier, the work of Nachemson[20] has shown that only in the horizontal position is the disc free of significant stress. The sitting position places substantial burden upon the lumbar disc; therefore, patients should be clearly informed that sitting at a desk or in an armchair does not provide adequate relief from stress on the lumbar spine.

Traction

Traction is a popular nonstandardized conservative treatment modality for low back pain and sciatica that has been used over the centuries. The principle behind it is the unloading of the spine by stretching muscles and ligaments and eventually significantly decreasing the intradiscal pressures. This goal, however, is not easily achieved. Nachemson and Elfstrom[21] concluded that a distraction force equivalent to 60 per cent of body weight is necessary to reduce intradiscal pressure at L3 only 25 per cent when the patient is standing. Moreover, even in the supine posture, a reduction of only 20 to 30 per cent of intradiscal pressure can be accomplished when as much as 30 kilos of traction is applied for three seconds.[21] Since the discs are prestressed owing to the advantageous position of the posterior ligaments of the spine,[22] zero intradiscal pressures have not been realized with actual traction.

The methodological limitations and the clinical and empirical acceptance of this treatment modality have led to double-blind studies examining the effects of traction on patients suffering from sciatica.[23, 24] No significant statistical differences were appreciated in terms of relief of symptoms between the groups receiving real traction and those with nonfunctional traction. Furthermore, Weber[23] found that traction had no effect on spinal mobility, tension signs, deep tendon reflexes, paresis, sensory deficit, or consumption of analgesics. In some cases, traction might not only accomplish little amelioration of symptoms but may actually aggravate symptoms,[7] although the modality is usually well tolerated.

The use of traction, however, should not be totally discredited. Weber[23] appreciated a positive psychologic effect as to the patient's expectations for recovery while in traction. The authors, however, have found that traction is occasionally helpful in enforcing a prescription of bed rest, which is the most important facet of conservative management.

Manipulation

Empiricism has also fostered popularity of the use of spinal manipulation as a conservative modality in treating the low back pain syndrome. The principle behind its use is based on the assumption that subluxation of the vertebra precipitates low back complaints and that these complaints can be reduced with correction of the "misalignment." There is, however, "no scientific proof for or against either the efficacy of this spinal manipulation therapy or the pathophysiological foundation from which it is derived."[2]

Separate randomized studies in England that were designed to evaluate the efficacy of spinal manipulation therapy when compared with other conservative modalities failed to demonstrate any significant difference at one and three weeks after treatment.[6, 10] It was of interest, however, that a more rapid relief of pain was realized with manipulative therapy. Kirkaldy-Willis and Hull[16] have also found manipulation to be effective in well-defined posterior facet and sacroiliac joint syndromes.

Manipulative reduction of small disc protrusions has been reported,[5, 19] and reductions in the severity of the straight leg raising tension have also been demonstrated, but much skepticism remains.[3]

Grieve[11] has hypothesized the following mechanism that may contribute to the short term effects of manipulation: (1) relief of pain by an inhibitory effect on afferent painful stimuli, (2) relief of muscle spasm, (3) effect on tissue fluid exchange in collagenous tissue, (4) restoration of movement, and (5) placebo effect.

At this point, however, there are no scientific data to support the use of manipulation on a regular basis with low back pain or sciatica secondary to degenerative disc disease. It has not been shown to shorten the course of symptomatic disc disease or to lessen the morbidity. In cases of pathologic bone disease involving the lumbosacral spine, manipulation may be harmful.

Flexion Exercises

Lumbar flexion exercise becomes important in the subacute or chronic phases of lumbar disc degeneration (Fig. 4–2). The use of lumbar flexion exercises is based on the theory expounded by Williams.[31] The overall aim is to reduce the lumbar lordosis. The reversal of the lumbar curve and full flexion of the lumbosacral joint will accomplish this goal. Subluxed overriding facet joints are placed in a position where they no longer overlap. Second, the spine is placed in a position of greater stability where the shearing stresses are minimized at the lower lumbar levels. Third, the intervertebral foramina are widened, allowing maximum room for exit of the nerve roots. A fourth goal of lumbar flexion exercises is to strengthen the abdominal musculature and the flexors of the spine. Both of these muscle groups have been shown to be important in supporting the spine and alleviating stress on the intervertebral disc. All of these goals and the reasons for the effectiveness of a lumbar flexion exercise program are open to question. Their efficacy, however, on an empirical and clinical basis has

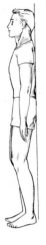

Lumbar spine exercises.

Two exercise sessions every day: (Morning and night *OR* afternoon and night).

Start with two (2) of each and gradually increase to ten (10) of each (twice a day), over a period of 10 days to two weeks.

1. Stand with back against wall and heels flat on the floor. Flatten "small" of back against wall by rotating pelvis up and forward.

   NOTE: No space between small of back and wall.

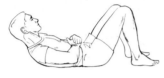

2. Lie on back with knees bent and feet flat on floor. Place hands on abdomen. Raise head and upper part of spinal column while contracting abdominal muscles.

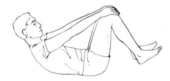

3. Lie on back. Separate legs. Bend knees and hips, and draw knees up toward axillae by clasping them with hands. *NOT TO BE DONE BY POSTOPERATIVE SPINE FUSION PATIENTS.*

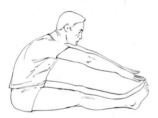

4. Sit on floor with legs outstretched. Touch toes without bending knees. When able to touch toes, stretch beyond toes. "Spring."

5. Lie flat on back. Without bending knees, lift one leg straight up, bending at hip; then the other; then both together.

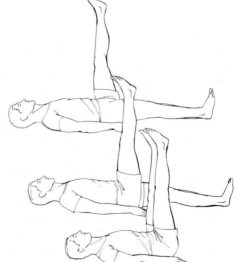

Figure 4–2. Lumbar spine exercises. (From Rothman, R. H., and Simeone, F. A.: The Spine, 2nd ed. Philadelphia, W. B. Saunders Co., 1982.)

been clearly shown. Recently, isometric lumbar flexion exercises have shown promise.

Lumbar flexion exercise should not be instituted in acute disc hernia-tion until the patient's symptoms have subsided to the point at which list and paravertebral muscle spasm are no longer noted and the major part of the acute symptomatology has subsided. This will usually be two to three weeks after the initiation of conservative therapy. Gentle exercises are started, being immediately discontinued if a flare-up of the patient's symptomatology appears. The exercises may be reinstituted at a later date when the patient's tolerance for them has increased. It is not necessary, however, to wait until the patient is asymptomatic before instituting this program of exercise.

General Measures of Back Hygiene – The Low Back School

Along with a program of lumbar flexion exercises, the patient with lumbar disc degeneration should be educated in certain measures of back hygiene that are in accord with the flexion management of these disorders. He should be instructed to sleep on his side or back with his legs and hips in a position of flexion and should be cautioned against the prone position, which hyperextends the lumbar spine. This is particularly true in spinal stenosis. If the patient is in a hospital bed, the Fowler position should be utilized. When the individual is sitting in a chair, he should sit with the buttocks well forward and the spine in a flexed position. This position is sometimes referred to as "slumping" and is regarded with a sense of horror by many physical therapists. It is our feeling, however, that people will habitually assume this situation because of the comfort it provides. Cross-ing the legs while seated will add further flexion to this position and is also desirable.

Lifting heavy loads above the waist should be prohibited, particularly those in which the patient is forced to rock back into a position of hyperextension. When picking up a load from the floor, the patient must be cautioned to utilize the musculature of his legs and bend from the knee and hip, rather than the thoracic and lumbar spine. It is most important, however, that the length of the lever arm (the distance between the lumbar spine and the object being lifted) used during lifting be kept at a mini-mum.[26]

Although most patients can be instructed on the prophylactic aspects of back hygiene on an office visit, a structured, multifaceted approach has been designed particularly for the chronic and subacute low back pain patient. The concept of the Back School was conceived by Zackissen-Forcel, a physiotherapist at the Danderyd Hospital in Sweden in 1970.[28, 33] The audio-visual program that evolved had as its data base the currently appreciated anatomic, epidemiologic, and biomechanical factors that give rise to low back pain.

Initially, the patient is introduced to the goals of the Back School and to the anatomy and physiology that contribute to the development of back disorders. The various treatment modalities that are described emphasize natural healing processes that, if allowed, would lead to the amelioration of symptoms.

The patient is then instructed in the applied biomechanics of the spine and in how posture analysis can allow one to reduce the forces that come to bear on the lumbar spine and precipitate symptoms. Muscle function, particularly of the abdomen, is emphasized as the intrinsic dynamic support that one can actively utilize to improve low back function.

The final goal of the program is to emphasize that back hygiene can be most effectively realized if the patient remains physically and socially active in his environment despite the apparent physical handicap. Thus far, this multifaceted approach has yielded more encouraging results than routine physiotherapeutic modalities.[7]

Physical Therapy

The use of local heat and light massage are well tolerated and pleasant for most patients with low back syndrome, but aside from their relaxing capabilities, they add little to the efficacy of bed rest alone.

Braces and Corsets

Routine immobilization of the lumbar spine will rapidly lead to soft tissue contracture and muscle atrophy. For this reason, the use of rigid lumbar braces is seldom recommended. The young patient with degenerative disease is more advantageously treated with a program designed to increase his range of motion and strengthen his musculature rather than one based upon immobilization.

There are, however, certain instances in which the external support plays a useful role. The obese patient with poor abdominal musculature is frequently fitted with a firm corset with flexible metal stays (Fig. 4–3). This corset serves the function of reinforcing the abdominal musculature and thereby increases the patient's efficiency in utilizing the thoracic and abdominal cavities to support and extend the spine.[29] Nachemson and Morris[30] demonstrated that the support realized with the lumbosacral corset is reflected in the diminution of intradiscal pressure by approximately 30 per cent.

The mechanism whereby the thoracic and abdominal cavities act as extensions of the spine is discussed in Chapter I, Anatomy of the Spine. It would be preferable, of course, to train these patients to develop their abdominal musculature and shed unnecessary adipose tissue.

A second category of individuals for whom braces are utilized are elderly individuals with advanced multilevel degenerative changes. These patients will not tolerate an exercise program, and indeed, their symptomatology is frequently intensified by a program of mobilization. Depending on the extent of their disease, a Knight-Taylor brace with shoulder straps

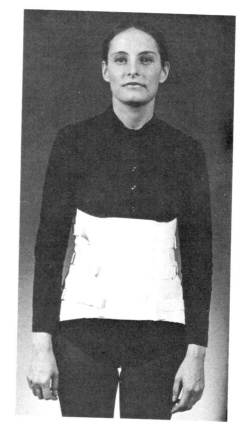

Figure 4–3. The lumbosacral corset with flexible metal stays utilized for abdominal and spinal support. (From Rothman, R. H., and Simeone, F. A.: The Spine, 2nd ed. Philadelphia, W. B. Saunders Co., 1982.)

or possibly a short lumbosacral brace with rigid metal stays is used to partially immobilize the spine and place the arthritic joints at rest (Fig. 4–4). With bracing, marked relief of pain is rapidly achieved in these individuals. Frequently, it is possible to wean these people from their support, which should be attempted, if possible, after their acute symptoms subside. This is to prevent further loss of muscle tone and stiffness in an already weakened spine.

Bracing is no longer employed in the postoperative management of patients who have undergone spine fusion. If more than a two-level spinal fusion is undertaken (i.e., L3 to the sacrum or longer), the brace may be utilized.

Pregnancy and Lumbar Disc Problems

One of the most challenging problems confronting the orthopedic surgeon is the pregnant patient presenting with symptoms of disc degeneration. It is our feeling that the intervertebral disc is placed under excessive stress during pregnancy for two reasons. The first reason is the obvious extra burden of carrying the fetus, and the second is the unusual ligamentous laxity found during pregnancy. The laxity is caused by maternal production of relaxin and relaxin-like hormones. Relaxin is a

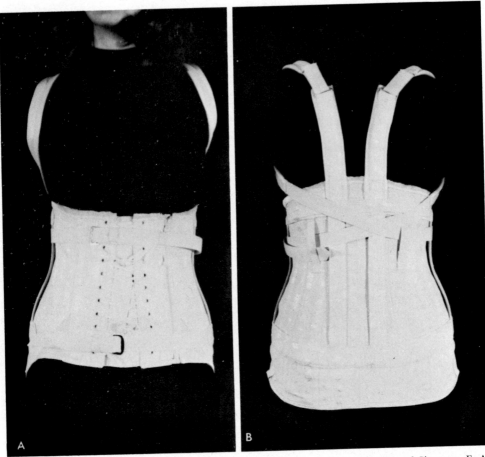

Figure 4–4. Knight-Taylor brace; *A*, front, *B*, back. (From Rothman, R. H., and Simeone, F. A.: *The Spine*, 2nd ed. Philadelphia, W. B. Saunders Co., 1982.)

hormone found in many mammals that produces the ligamentous laxity about the pelvis necessary for the birth of offspring that may be larger than the bony pelvic outlet. It is possible that a similar hormome produced near term in humans may contribute to the development of congenital hip dislocation and can certainly be of importance in producing relaxation of the ligamentous supporting structures of the spine.

The therapeutic modalities available during pregnancy are somewhat limited. For the most part, one must depend upon bed rest and the use of a supporting corset, although the latter is frequently very uncomfortable. A very well tolerated alternative is a century-old supporting corset that has been used by Japanese women during the latter months of pregnancy. The "Iwata-Obi" is a Japanese maternity support that is made up of approximately five yards of eight inch cotton cloth, with the lateral third being made of soft elastic material. The terminal four inches of cotton are tapered to allow for easy tucking or pinning after it has been wrapped around the lower abdomen to provide greater support. Empirically, this device seems to increase the abdominal support that has been lost by the attenuated muscle fibers, particularly in the latter months of pregnancy.[27]

The physician hesitates to prescribe potent and potentially teratogenic drugs during pregnancy. Diagnosis is also somewhat hampered by the limited use of x-ray during the first trimester of pregnancy. Surgery, of course, is the last resort during pregnancy and is indicated only in the presence of serious neurologic findings. It is often necessary to prescribe long periods of bed rest for a pregnant patient in order for her to obtain a measure of relief. The use of a firm, flexible corset or the Japanese modification is of great help in relieving the spine of excessive stress.

DRUG THERAPY

The intelligent use of drug therapy is an important modality in the treatment of lumbar disc disease. Three categories of pharmacologic agents are utilized: (1) anti-inflammatory drugs, (2) analgesics, and (3) muscle relaxants. Both mechanical compression of neural structures and inflammatory reaction contribute to the symptoms of low back pain and sciatica. The inflammatory reaction is most likely the result of the local irritant sequela of nerve compression as well as the poorly understood autoimmune phenomenon (see section on Clinical Syndromes).

Gertzbein and others[35] have summarized the following clinical observations that support the contention that an inflammatory reaction contributes to the pathogenesis of the various degenerative disc syndromes:

1. In entrapment syndromes, the predominant features are numbness and paresthesia as opposed to pain, which is predominantly a feature of inflammation.

2. The findings at surgery are compatible with perineural inflammation and, in a later stage, perineural fibrosis.

3. The microscopic picture of vascular ingrowth, granulation, and fibrosis in degenerative discs is compatible with an inflammatory reaction.

4. Dramatic relief is reported in patients who are treated with local or systemic anti-inflammatory drugs.

Several double-blind studies have compared various anti-inflammatory drugs in the treatment of low back pain with or without sciatica, and generally, no difference in their efficacy was demonstrated.[34, 37, 38, 41, 42] Most of these studies, however, do not quantify the contributing beneficial effects of bed rest prescribed along with the various medications. Wiesel and Rothman[42] concluded that aspirin or phenylbutazone (Butazolidin) in conjunction with bed rest were no more effective in relieving symptoms of acute lumbago than bed rest with the non-anti-inflammatory acetaminophen. Green,[36] however, found that initially high but tapering doses of the steroid dexamethasone were beneficial in the treatment of sciatica from myelographically proven disc hernia that had failed to respond to bed rest alone.

In principle, the authors feel that anti-inflammatory medication, particularly in the form of aspirin, 10 to 15 grains every four hours, should be utilized in conjunction with bed rest for treatment of low back pain due to disc disease with sciatica. In those individuals with gastrointestinal intolerance, buffered or enteric-coated aspirin or the liquid methyl salicylate can safely be used.

It has been the authors' experience, as well as others',[36, 40] that certain patients who fail to show a response to aspirin may obtain dramatic relief from a short course of systemic steroids. This can be done either in the hospital or at home, as long as the patient is aware that he must strictly adhere to the prescription instructions. The dosages of dexamethasone prescribed are 6 mg. four times on day 1, 4 mg. four times on day 2, 2 mg. four times on day 3, 1 mg. three times on day 4, 0.75 mg. twice on day 5, 0.5 mg. twice on day 6, and 0.5 mg. once on day 7. This regimen has been well tolerated even in patients with a history of peptic ulcer disease and diabetes, if used with appropriate precautions.

As their acute disc symptoms are resolved, patients may have residual chronic symptomatology of low back pain that will require anti-inflammatory medications, usually in lower doses than those used for the acute lesions.

The judicious use of analgesics is of extreme importance during the acute phase of disc disease. It is our feeling that if pain is of such severe nature that parenteral narcotics are required, morphine sulfate is the drug of choice. The dosage should be adequate to provide substantial relief of the patient's symptoms. Patients must be reassured that pain medication is available for their use and that a stoic attitude is therefore not essential. Many times during the acute early phases of treatment, the narcotics will be ordered on a regular basis rather than as the patient requests them. This will relieve the patient of the burden of summoning and waiting for nurses to obtain pain medication. Constipation is an untoward side-effect of many of the opiates, and a stool softener should be added to the regimen if prolonged use of narcotics is required. As pain subsides, oral codeine or non-narcotic analgesics may be substituted for more potent drugs.

The authors infrequently use muscle relaxants, which may be effective at times in acute disc lesions in which muscle spasm is a prominent finding. Methocarbamol and carisoprodol are the drugs most commonly used for this purpose. Either of them may cause drowsiness. Carisoprodol is administered in a dosage of 350 mg. two times daily; the dosage for methocarbamol is 1.5 gm. four times daily. Occasionally, in an extremely acute problem of marked paravertebral muscle spasm, therapy will be initiated with the use of 10 ml. of intravenous methocarbamol, which is later continued with the oral form of the drug. This will frequently produce striking relief of both pain and limitation of motion. Muscle relaxants are rarely used in the chronic or subacute phase of disc degeneration.

It has been found of value to add a sedative or mild tranquilizer to the patient's regimen to alleviate any anxiety and make a prolonged period of bed rest more tolerable. Phenobarbital in 15 to 30 mg. doses four times daily will accomplish this goal. The use of diazepam in chronic and acute low back pain as either a muscle relaxant or tranquilizer should be discouraged,[39] since it is actually a depressant and will accentuate the depression that is often an integral feature of an individual's symptom complex. By contrast, the cautious use of antidepressants such as amitriptyline or thioridazine is often of great help in the depressed patient who expresses his inner conflict as low back pain.

REFERENCES

GENERAL

1. Anderson, B. J. G., and Ortegren, R.: Myoelectric back muscle activity during sitting. Scand. J. Rehab. Med. (Suppl. *3*):73, 1974.
2. Anonymous: The Scientific Status of the Fundamentals of Chiropractic: Analysis and Recommendations. National Institute of Neurological and Communicative Disorders and Stroke. April 8, 1975.
3. Chrisman, O. D., Mattracht, A., and Snook, G. A.: A study of the results following rotatory manipulation in the lumbar intervertebral disc syndrome. J. Bone Joint Surg., *46A*:517, 1964.
4. Colonna, P. C., and Friedenberg, Z.: The disc syndrome. J. Bone Joint Surg., *31A*:614, 1949.
5. Cyriax, J.: Dural pain. Lancet, *1*:919, 1978.
6. Doran, D. M., and Newell, D. J.: Manipulation in treatment of low back pain. A multi-center study. Br. Med. J., *1*:161, 1975.
7. Eie, N., and Kristiansen, K.: Komplikasjouer os Farer sed Tzakljoulehandling av Lumbale Skiveprolape. T. Morkse Loejeforen, *81*:1517, 1961.
8. Finnegan, W., Rothman, R. H., et al.: Results of surgical intervention in the symptomatic multiply-operated back patient. J. Bone Joint Surg., *61A/7*:1077, 1979.
9. Fink, J. W.: The straight leg raising test. Its relevance to possible disc pathology. N. Z. Med. J., *81*:557, 1975.
10. Glover, J. R., Morris, J. G., and Khosla, T.: Back pain: a randomized clinical trial of rotational manipulation of the trunk. Br. J. Ind. Med., *31*:59, 1974.
11. Grieve, G. P.: Manipulation. Physiotherapy, *61*:11, 1975.
12. Hakelius, A.: Prognosis in sciatica. Acta Orthop. Scand., *129*:6, 1970.
13. Henderson, R. S.: The treatment of lumbar intervertebral disc protrusion. Br. Med. J., *2*:597, 1952.
14. Herkowitz, H. N., Wiesel, S. W., Booth, R. E., Jr., and Rothman, R. H.: Metrizamide myelography and epidural venography: their role in the diagnosis of lumbar disc herniation and spinal stenosis. In Press.
15. Key, J. A.: The conservative and operative treatment of lesions of the intervertebral discs in the low back. Surgery, *17*:291, 1945.
16. Kikaldy-Willis, W. M., and Hill, R. J.: A more precise diagnosis for low back pain. Spine, *4* #1:102, 1979.
17. Marshall, L. L.: Conservative management of low back pain: a review of 700 cases. Med. J. Aust. *1*:266, 1967.
18. Mathews, J. A., and Hickling, J.: Lumbar traction: a double-bind controlled study for sciatica. Rheum. Rehab., *14*:222, 1975.
19. Mathews, J. A., and Yater, D. A. H.: Reduction of lumbar disc prolapse by manipulation. Br. Med. J., *3*:696, 1969.
20. Nachemson, A.: The load on lumbar disks indifferent positions of the body. Acta Orthop. Scand., *36*:426, 1965.
21. Nachemson, A., and Elfstrom, G.: Intravital dynamic pressure measurements in lumbar disc. Scan. J. Rehab. Med. (Suppl. *1*):5, 1970.
22. Nachemson, A.: Rheumatology and Rheumatism. In Press. 1981.
23. Weber, H.: Lumbar disc herniation. A prospective study of prognostic factors including a controlled trial. Part I. J. Oslo City Hosp., 28:36, 1978.
24. Weber, H.: Traction therapy in sciatica due to disc prolapse. J. Oslo City Hosp., *23*:167, 1973.
25. Wiesel, S. W., and Rothman, R. H.: Acute low back pain. An objective analysis of conservative therapy. Spine, *5*:324, 1980.

FLEXION EXERCISES

26. Anderson, G. B. J., Ortengren, R., and Nachemson, A.: Quantitative study of back loads in lifting. Spine. 1(3):178, 1976.
27. Hecter, A. W., Budd, F. W., and Curlin, J. P.: "IWATA Obi" (Japanese Maternity Lumbosacral Support). Milit. Med., 24:359, 1972.
28. Lidstrom, A., and Zachrissen, M.: Physical therapy on low back pain and sciatica. An attempt at evaluation. Scand. J. Rehab. Med., 2:37, 1970.
29. Morris, J. M.: Low back bracing. Clin. Orthop., 102:120, 1974.
30. Nachemson, A., and Morris, J. M.: In vivo measurements of intradiscal pressure: Discometry, a method for determination of pressure in the lower lumbar disc. J. Bone Joint Surg.. 46A:1077, 1964.
31. Williams, R. C.: Examination and conservative treatment for disc lesions of the lower spine. Clin. Orthop., 5:28, 1955.
32. Williams, S. J.: Back School. Physiotherapy, 63:590, 1977.
33. Zachrissen, M.: The Low Back Pain School. Danderyd's Hospital, Danderyd, Sweden, 1972.

DRUG THERAPY

34. Barretter, R. R.: A double blind comparative study of carisprodol, propoxyphene and placebo in the mangement of low back syndromes. Curr. Therap. Res., 20:233, 1976.
35. Gertzbein, S. D., Tile, M., Gross, A., and Falk, R.: Autoimmunity and degenerative disc disease of the lumbar spine. Orthop. Clin. North Am., 6:67, 1975.
36. Green, L. N.: Dexamethasone on the management of symptoms due to herniated lumbar disc. J. Neurol. Neurosurg. Psychiat., 38:1211, 1975.
37. Hingorani, K., and Templeton, J. S.: A comparative trial of azapropazone and ketoprofen in the treatment of acute backache. Curr. Med. Res. Opin., 3:407, 1975.
38. Jaffe, G.: A double blind multi-center comparison of naproxen and indomethacin in acute musculoskeletal disorders. Current Med. Res. Opinion, 4:373, 1976.
39. Mooney, V., and Cairns, D.: Management of patient with chronic low back pain. Orthop. Clin. North Am., 9:543, 1978.
40. Naylor, A., and Turner, R.: ACTH in treatment of lumbar disc prolapse. Proc. Royal Soc. Med., 54:15, 1961.
41. Vignon, G.: Comparative study of intravenous ketoprofen versus aspirin. Rheum. Rehab., 15:83, 1976.
42. Wiesel, S. W., and Rothman, R. H.: Acute low back pain, an objective analysis of conservative therapy. Spine, 5:324, 1980.

Chapter 5

"SALVAGE" LUMBAR SPINE SURGERY

INTRODUCTION

The evaluation and treatment of the patient with previous lumbar spine surgery are becoming increasing problems. There are approximately 300,000 de novo laminectomies performed each year in the United States, and it is estimated that 15 per cent of these patients will continue to have significant disability.[14] The inherent complexity of these patients demands a method of problem-solving that is precise and unambiguous.

The best solution for preventing recurrent low back pain after lumbar spine surgery would be to prevent the problem from occurring. This emphasizes the point that proper surgical indications for the initial procedure should be strictly followed.[8, 12, 24] The idea of "exploring" the low back when no objective criteria are present is no longer acceptable. In fact, even when hard findings are present and the patient is psychologically unstable or there are compensation-litigation factors, the outcome of low back surgery is uncertain.[20] Thus, the initial decision to operate is the most important one. Once the situation of recurrent pain after surgery is created, the potential for a solution is limited at best.

The situation confronting the physician is to distinguish the patient with a mechanical lesion from the patient whose symptoms are secondary to a nonmechanical problem. The types of mechanical lesion include recurrent herniated disc, spinal instability, and spinal stenosis. These three entities produce symptoms on a nerve pressure basis and are amenable to surgical intervention. The nonmechanical lesions consist of scar tissue, whether it be arachnoiditis or perineural fibrosis, psychosocial instability, or a medical disease. These problems will not be helped by additional lumbar spine surgery.

The keystone for successful treatment is to obtain an accurate diagnosis. Although a seemingly obvious need, this essential step is often not taken. Consequently, the rehabilitation of this patient group has been fraught with difficulty. The goals of this chapter are to analyze the major points in the "work-up" of the multiply operated back patient, to discuss each of the mechanical lesions, and to review the technique of revision spine surgery.

EVALUATION

Each patient who has undergone a previous lumbar spine operation seems to have a unique and involved history. These people often want to relate their entire story to the evaluating physician, and it is best to let them do so. However, there are several important points in the patient's history that are necessary in the decision-making process in order to arrive at a diagnosis, and these should be specifically sought. First, it should be determined that the discomfort of these patients is not based on non-orthopedic causes such as pancreatitis or abdominal aneurysm. If there is any question, a thorough medical evaluation should be obtained and the individuals should be appropriately treated. In addition, if there is any indication of psychosocial instability, as evidenced by alcoholism, drug dependence, depression, or litigious involvement, a thorough psychiatric evaluation is necessary. It has been clearly demonstrated that persons with profound emotional disturbance and those in the midst of active litigation do not derive observable benefit from any further surgery.[19] In many cases, once a patient's underlying psychosocial problem has been successfully treated, the somatic back complaints and disability will disappear.

Once it is determined that the lumbar spine is the probable source of the patient's complaints, three specific historical points need clarification. The first factor is the number of previous lumbar spine operations. It has been shown by Waddell and coworkers[22] in Canada and Finnigan and colleagues[5] in the United States that with every subsequent lumbar spine operation, the percentage of good results decreases. Statistically, the second operation has a 50 per cent chance of success, and beyond two operations, patients are more likely to be made worse than to be helped.

The next important historical point to determine is the pain-free interval that the patient obtained from his previous operation. If the patient awakes from surgery and his pain is still present, the nerve root may not have been properly decompressed, the wrong level may have been explored, or the disc may not have been completely excised. If the pain-free interval is greater than six months, the patient may have pain on the basis of a herniated disc at the same level or at a different level. If, however, the pain-free interval is between one month and six months, the diagnosis is most often arachnoiditis.[5]

Finally, the patient's pain pattern is evaluated. If leg pain predominates, a herniated disc or spinal stenosis is most likely. If back pain predominates, instability, tumor, infection, or arachnoiditis are the major considerations. If both back and leg pain are present, spinal stenosis or arachnoiditis are the possibilities.

Physical examination is the next major step in the evaluation of the multiply operated back patient. The neurologic examination and a tension sign such as the straight leg raising test or the sitting root test are noted. It is most helpful to have the results of a dependable previous examination so that a comparison can be made. If the neurologic picture is unchanged from before the previous surgery and the tension signs are negative, mechanical compression is unlikely. However, if there is a new neurologic deficit or the tension signs are positive, pressure on the neural elements is possible.

Roentgenographic studies are the last major part of the patient's work-up. Again, it is most helpful to have a previous set of plain x-rays and a myelogram for comparison. The extent and level of previous laminectomies and evidence of spinal stenosis are evaluated on the plain roentgenograms. Lateral flexion/extension x-rays of the lumbar spine are examined to see if instability is present. An unstable spine may be the result of the patient's intrinsic disease or secondary to a previous surgical procedure.

Computerized axial tomography (CAT) is employed if there is any question of spinal stenosis. In many instances, the patient will have subjective symptoms but not objective findings. When leg pain is a major complaint, the CAT scan is most useful. Bony encroachment in the lateral recesses and foramina can be specifically evaluated with this study. As the technology of the CAT scan advances, the technique will be used to study not only the osseous structures in relation to the neural elements but the soft tissue components such as the intervertebral discs and ligaments as well.

Contrast studies are reserved for those patients who have either a new neurologic deficit or a positive tension sign. Also, preoperative patients with a diagnosis of spinal stenosis or spinal instability will undergo a myelogram to make sure that there are no additional pathologic features. Pain in and of itself is an inadequate justification for myelography. Metrizamide, a water-soluble contrast agent, is now employed when the problem is confined to the lumbar spine and is very satisfactory in defining neural compression.

DIFFERENTIAL DIAGNOSIS

A specific diagnosis is necessary if an additional operation on the spine is to succeed. Basically, the physician is trying to separate the patients whose symptoms are on a mechanical basis from the patients who have pain secondary to scar tissue. It should be appreciated that although this discussion is oriented toward the surgical salvage of lumbar spine patients, the authors do not wish to imply that nothing can be accomplished with nonoperative measures. Epidural steroids, transcutaneous nerve stimulation, facet rhizolysis, operant conditioning, bracing, antidepressant medication, and patient education are some of the modalities that have been employed to deal with these problems.[1, 7, 10, 13, 15, 16, 21, 23] However, for the majority of patients, these treatment regimens are at best palliative and frequently offer only short-term solutions.

When a patient first arrives at the multiply operated back clinic, an information form is completed, as shown in Figure 5-1. This is most important, for, at best, these patients are difficult to evaluate, and if the information is obtained in an organized manner, there is less chance of something being missed. For a patient to be evaluated, a physician's or hospital summary form and the x-rays and myelograms (*not* reports) completed before the initial and most recent surgery must be obtained. This information is invaluable in the decision-making process, for in many cases one will find that the initial operation was not indicated.

THE MULTIPLY OPERATED BACK

Name_____ Age_____ Date_____

Weight_____ Height _____ Social Security No._____

II. History:
    A. Number of back operations_____
    B. First operation: Date _____
        1. Pre-operative Complaints: Back Pain_____ Leg Pain_____ Combined_____
        2. Pain-free interval after first operation: None_____ Up to 4 Weeks_____
           One month to one year_____ Greater than one year_____
        3. Review of physician's report: Neurologic Exam_____
                                    Straight Leg Raising Test_____
        4. Review of first pre-operative myelogram (Type)_____
    C. Last Operation: Date_____
        1. Pre-operative complaints: Back Pain_____ Leg Pain _____ Combined_____
        2. Pain-free interval after last operation: None_____ Up to 4 weeks_____
           One month to one year_____ Greater than one year_____
        3. Review of physician's report: Neurologic Exam_____
                                    Straight Leg Raising Test_____
        4. Review of last pre-operative myelogram (Type)_____
    D. Present complaints: Back Pain_____ Leg Pain_____ Combined_____

III. Physical Exam
    A. Back: Range of Motion (%)_____ Point Tenderness_____
    B. Neurologic Exam: Knee Jerk_____ Ankle Jerk_____ Quadriceps Weakness_____
                E.H.L. Weakness_____
    C. Straight Leg Raising_____ Crossed SLR_____

IV. X-rays:
    Plain_____ Motion_____ Bone Scan_____ CAT Scan_____
    Myelogram (Type)_____

V. Medical/GYN Evaluation

VI. Psycho-social Assessment: Divorce_____ Alcohol_____ Drugs_____
    Multiple Jobs_____ Depression_____ Compensation_____ Litigation_____

VII. Diagnosis: HNP (Level)   Spinal Stenosis   Spinal Instability
              Arachnoiditis   Other

VIII. Treatment Plan

Figure 5–1. Sample patient information form.

Table 5–1 is a summary of the various pathologic entities and the signs and symptoms that need to be considered in these patients. Figure 5–2 is a graphic display using the information from Table 5–1. Each of the pathologic problems that respond to surgery can be differentiated from arachnoiditis, which is not amenable to an operation. It must be stressed that the incidence of surgical problems is many times lower than that of scar tissue.

TABLE 5–1. Differential Diagnosis of the Multiply Operated Back

History-Physical Radiographs	Original Disc Not Removed	Recurrent Disc At Same Level	Recurrent Disc At Different Level	Spinal Instability	Spinal Stenosis	Arachnoiditis
# Previous Operations						>1
Pain-Free Interval	None	>6 months	>6 months			>1 month but <6 months
Predominant Pain (Leg Versus Back)	Leg Pain	Leg Pain	Leg Pain	Back Pain	Back and Leg Pain	Back and Leg Pain
Tension Sign	+	+	+			
Neurologic Exam	+ Same Pattern	+ Same Pattern	+ Different Level			May Be Positive
Plain X-rays	+ If Wrong Level				+	
Lateral Motion X-rays				+ after Stress		
Metrizamide Myelogram	+ But Unchanged	+ Same Level	+ Different Level		+	+
C.A.T. Scan		+ Same Level	+ Different Level		+	

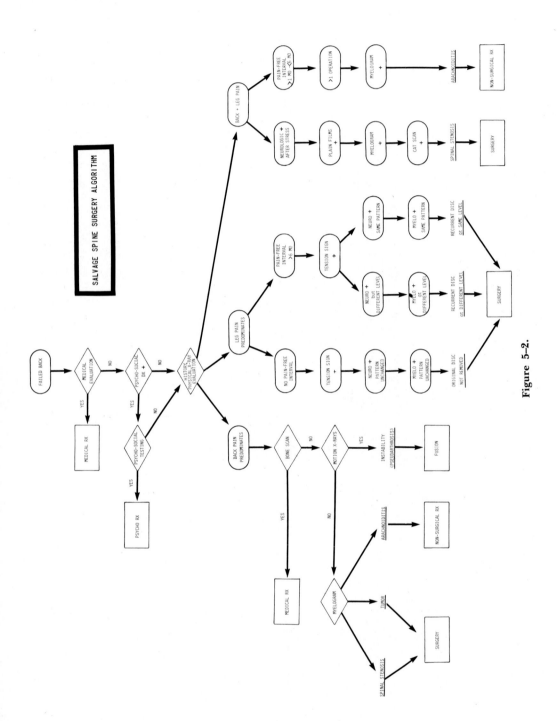

Figure 5–2.

Figure 5–3. Wrong level decompressed. *A*, Laminotomy at L5–S1 (arrow)—patient continued to have complaints. *B*, Original myelogram shows defect one level higher at L4–L5.

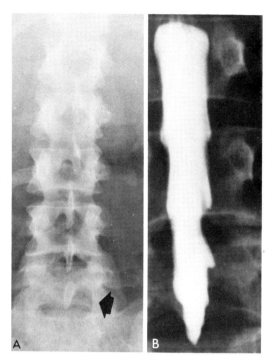

Herniated Intervertebral Disc

Three possibilities exist if the patient's pain is based on a herniated disc. First, the original disc may not have been satisfactorily removed. The wrong level may have been decompressed, the laminectomy that was performed may not have been wide enough, or a fragment of disc material may have been left behind (Fig. 5–3). These patients will have predominant leg pain, and the neurologic examination, tension sign, and myelographic pattern will remain unchanged from the preoperative state. The differentiating feature is that these patients will have no pain-free interval. They will wake up from the operation complaining of their preoperative pain. These patients will be aided by a technically correct laminectomy.

A second possibility is that there is a recurrent herniated intervertebral disc at the previously decompressed level (Fig. 5–4). These patients complain of sciatica and have an unchanged neurologic examination, tension sign, and myelogram. The distinguishing characteristic of these patients is that their pain-free interval is greater than six months. Another operative procedure is indicated in patients with this clinical presentation.

Finally, a recurrent disc may occur at a different level. These patients will have a pain-free interval greater than six months; sciatica will predominate, and their tension signs will be positive. However, a neurologic deficit, if present, and the myelogram will be positive at a different level. In this situation, a repeat operation will yield beneficial results.

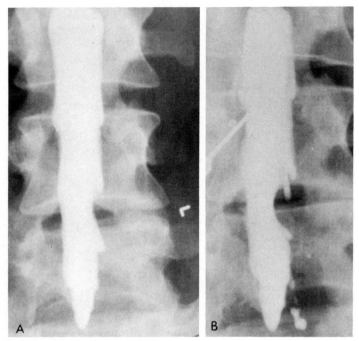

Figure 5–4. Recurrent disc at same level. *A*, Disc at L4–L5. Patient had good relief for 18 months. *B*, Recurrent leg pain. Myelogram demonstrates recurrent disc at same level.

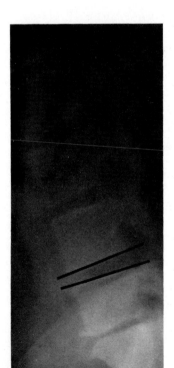

Figure 5–5. Flexion of lumbar spine demonstrating a reversal of normal lordotic curve at L4–L5.

Lumbar Instability

Lumbar instability is another major condition causing pain in the multiply operated back patient on a mechanical basis. The etiology may be from the patient's intrinsic back disease or an excessively wide bilateral laminectomy. Pseudoarthrosis is included in this category as it would be painful on the basis of the instability it would create. Patients with instability will complain predominantly of back pain, and their physical examination may be negative. The key to the diagnosis of these patients is

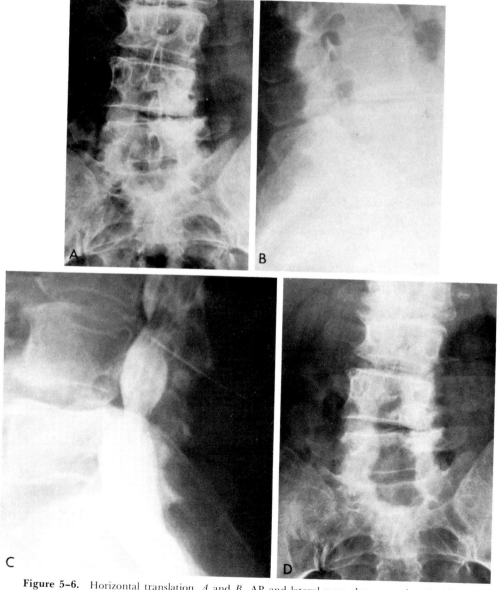

Figure 5–6. Horizontal translation. *A* and *B*, AP and lateral x-ray demonstrating significant degenerative changes in a 63-year-old. *C*, Myelogram with block at L4–L5. *D*, Postoperatively after midline decompression.

Illustration continued on following page

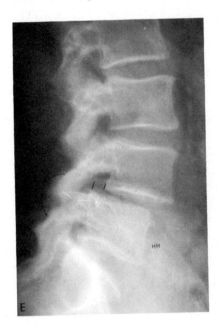

Figure 5–6 *Continued.* *E*, Two years later shows instability with a slip of L4 on L5.

the lateral flexion/extension x-rays. Reversal of the normal lordotic curve at a motion segment (Fig. 5–5) and anterior-posterior translation of one vertebral body on another (Fig. 5–6) are the radiographic criteria for diagnosing segmental instability and would constitute a strong indication for spinal fusion or repair of a pseudoarthrosis. Finally, the presence of a

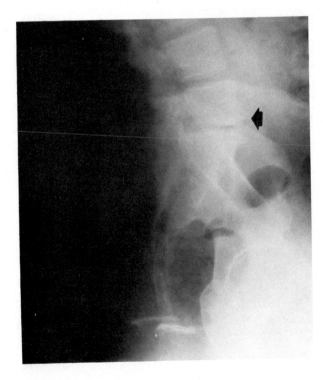

Figure 5–7. Traction osteophyte at the anterior inferior border of L5 (arrow). Indirect evidence of instability.

traction osteophyte (Fig. 5–7), as described by Ian MacNab, should alert the surgeon to the possible presence of spinal instability.[11]

Spinal Stenosis

Spinal stenosis is also a major diagnostic entity that can mechanically produce pain. These patients complain of both back and leg pain. Their physical examination is often inconclusive, although, following exercise, a neurologic deficit may occur. This latter phenomenon is termed a positive stress test. The plain x-rays can be suggestive, displaying facet degeneration, decreased interpedicular distance, decreased sagittal canal diameter, and disc degeneration. A computerized axial tomogram will demonstrate bony encroachment upon the neural elements (Fig. 5–8). This is especially helpful in evaluating the lateral recesses. At this time, a metrizamide myelogram is the most definitive test and will demonstrate a block or significant narrowing of the dye column at the involved level. It should be appreciated that spinal stenosis and arachnoiditis can coexist.[3] Currently, it is felt that if there is definite evidence of bony compression, a laminectomy is indicated. However, if there is scar tissue, the degree of pain relief a patient may anticipate is uncertain.

Arachnoiditis

Arachnoiditis as a postoperative occurrence constitutes an area of considerable concern to the spinal surgeon. At the present state of the art, there is no effective cure for symptomatic arachnoiditis.

Arachnoiditis is strictly defined as an inflammation of the pia-arachnoid membrane surrounding the spinal cord or cauda equina.[1] The condition may be present in varying degrees of severity, from mild thickening of the membranes to solid adhesions. The scarring may be severe enough to obliterate the subarachnoid space, which may block the flow of contrast agents.

Statistically, the histories of these patients will reveal more than one

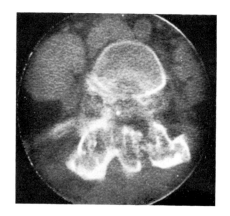

Figure 5–8. Computed axial tomogram (CAT) demonstrating postfusion spinal stenosis with compression of neural elements.

previous operation, and their pain-free interval will fall between one and six months. They may complain of both back and leg pain. The physical examination is not conclusive. The myelogram is definitive for the diagnosis, displaying nonvisualization of the nerve roots within the dural sac and narrowing or blockage of the contrast column at the involved levels (Fig. 5–9). There is no bony encroachment of the neural elements, since the symptoms originate from scar tissue formation.

Arachnoiditis is not amenable to surgical intervention, and nonsurgical modalities should be employed in its treatment. It should be emphasized that the diagnostic criteria to distinguish mechanical back pain from fibrosis are rarely as clearly defined as presented. As shown in Figure 5–2, a patient may have several positive signs for each diagnostic possibility; quite frequently, one or more of the findings may be missing in an individual patient, yet the patient still has pathology. For example, a patient who has pain secondary to a recurrent herniated disc at a different level may not have a positive neurologic examination. The sum of a patient's findings should help the physician in his diagnostic decision-making.

In conclusion, it needs to be stressed that the physician should take an organized approach in evaluating the multiply operated patient. The origin of the problem in the majority of patients is a faulty decision to perform the original procedure. Further surgery on the multiply operated back on an "exploratory" basis is not warranted and will lead only to further disability.[4] An additional operative procedure is indicated only when there are objective findings.

These patients need a total assessment. The etiology of each patient's complaint must be accurately localized and identified. In addition to the orthopedic evaluation, the patient's psychologic and general medical status

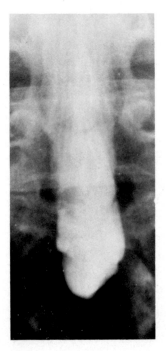

Figure 5–9. Arachnoiditis in multiply operated back patient. Metrizamide was used, but because of scar tissue, it looks as if Panopaque was employed.

need thorough investigation. Once the spine is identified as the source of the patient's symptoms, specific features should be sought in the patient's clinical history, physical examination, and radiographic evaluation. The number of previous operations, characteristics of the pain-free interval, and predominance of leg pain versus back pain are the major historical points. The neurologic examination and the presence of a tension sign are the important physical findings. Plain x-rays, motion films, metrizamide myelography, and computerized axial tomography have a specific place in the work-up. When all of the information is integrated, the physician can generally separate the patients with arachnoiditis from those with mechanical problems.

TECHNIQUE OF A REPEAT LAMINECTOMY

There are several technical aspects of performing a repeat laminectomy that require discussion. The goal of surgery is to relieve the neural elements of any mechanical pressure without violating the dura. The first difference from a de novo laminectomy is the operative approach. The surgeon cannot strip the paraspinal muscles with impunity because, at the previously operated sites, there will be no bone to protect the neural elements (Fig. 5–10). Thus, one must begin the approach at a new level to find the correct depth of the cauda equina, using a right-angle retractor and bovie to carefully extend the field over the unshielded area.

The surgeon may be tempted to try to remove the extradural scar tissue directly over the dura. Technically, this is quite difficult to perform, and there will be a great deal of hemorrhaging with a good possibility of injuring the dura. Additionally, even if the surgeon is successful in removing the scar tissue, there is no way of preventing its regrowth. Thus, the extradural scar tissue should be left alone.

It should be appreciated that the object of the surgical exercise is to visualize the lateral edge of the nerve roots. This is accomplished by extending the laminectomy from the new level down the lateral gutters, leaving the central scar tissue alone. Any bony encroachment or herniated disc material can then be easily removed.

Unfortunately, the risk of causing a dural tear is increased when a repeat laminectomy is performed, and the surgeon should be prepared to handle this complication. Each dural tear is different; however, certain basic principles should always be followed.

First, hemostasis should always be maintained so that if a dural tear occurs, the diagnosis can immediately be reached and the repair undertaken. A dural tear with a cerebrospinal fluid leak is very difficult to diagnose postoperatively. Radioiodinated serum albumin scans or myelograms can be diagnostic, but they are invasive procedures.[6, 9] However, there are no good noninvasive techniques available at the present time. Once a postoperative cerebrospinal fluid leak is diagnosed or highly suspected, the patient should quickly be taken to surgery to have the dura repaired. This is to prevent an infection in the cerebrospinal fluid.

The technique employed depends on the size and location of the dural

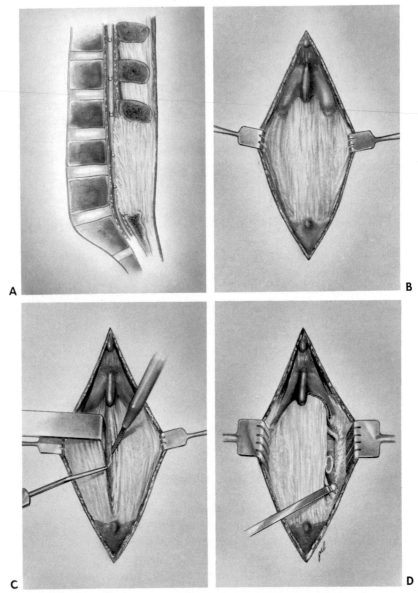

Figure 5–10. *A,* Lateral view showing that neural elements are unprotected at the previous operative site. *B,* View showing need to go to new level to appreciate depth of neural tissue. *C,* Bovie and retractor are carefully used to go laterally. *D,* Scar tissue over midline is left alone and nerve root with disc is exposed laterally.

tear (Fig. 5–11). For simple dural lacerations, 4-0 gauge silk sutures are used on a tapered or a reverse cutting with a one-half circle needle. A running locking suture or simple sutures incorporating a free fat graft give a watertight closure. When a large tear is present, a fascial graft (fascia lata for extra-large defects and lumbar fascia for small defects) can be used.[12] The grafts should be sutured in place with interrupted dural silk sutures. When a defect is in an inaccessible area, a small tissue plug of muscle or fat

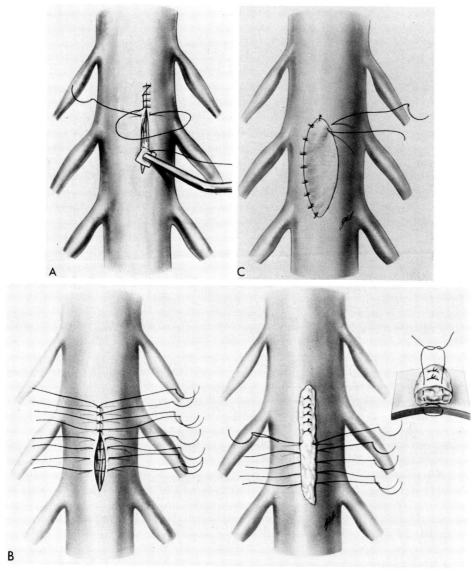

Figure 5–11. *A,* Dural repair with a running locking suture. *B,* Dural repair with interrupted sutures incorporating a free fat graft. *C,* Large dural tear repaired with a fascial graft. (From Eismont, F. J., et al.: Journal of Bone and Joint Surgery, in press, 1981.)

may be introduced through a second medial durotomy and pulled against the dural tear from inside the dura.[17]

Every repair should be tested by placing the patient in reverse Trendelenburg position and performing Valsalva maneuvers to increase the intrathecal pressure.

The fascia should be closed with a heavy nonabsorbable suture. The suture line should be watertight, and no drains should be used to prevent fistula formation should the dura leak later.

Postoperatively, the patient should be kept prone for five to seven days so that there is no increased pressure on the repair.

REFERENCES

1. Burton, C.: Lumbosacral arachnoiditis. Spine, *3*:24, 1978.
2. Coventry M. B., and Stauffer, R. N.: The multiply operated back. *In* American Academy of Orthopaedic Surgeons: Symposium on the Spine. St. Louis, C. V. Mosby, 1969, pp. 132–142.
3. Epstein, B. S.: The Spine. Philadelphia, Lea and Febiger, 1962.
4. Fager C. A., and Friedberg, S. R.: Analysis of failures and poor results of lumbar spine surgery. Spine, *5*:87, 1980.
5. Finnegan, W. J., Tenlin, J. M., Marvel, J. P., Nardine, R. J., and Rothman, R. H.: Results of surgical intervention in the symptomatic multiply-operated back patient. J. Bone Joint Surg., *61A*:1077, 1979.
6. Gass, H., Goldstein, A., Ruskin, R., and Leopold, N. A.: Chronic postmyelogram headache. Isotopic demonstration of dural leak and surgical care. Arch. Neurol., *25*:168, 1971.
7. Ghormley, R. K.: The problem of multiple operations on the back. *In* Edwards, J. W.: Instructional Course Lectures, Vol. 14. The American Academy of Orthopaedic Surgeons, Ann Arbor, 1957.
8. Hirsch, C.: Efficiency of surgery in low back disorders. J. Bone Joint Surg., *47A*:991, 1965.
9. Irjala, K., Suonpaa, J., and Laurent, B.: Identification of CSF leakage by immunofixation. Arch. Otolaryngol., *15*:447, 1979.
10. Loeser, J. D., Black, R. G., and Christman, A.: Relief of pain by transcutaneous stimulation. J. Neurosurg., *42*:308, 1975.
11. MacNab, I.: The traction spur. An indicator of segmental instability. J. Bone Joint Surg., *53A*:663, 1971.
12. Mayfield, F. H., and Kurokawa, K.: Watertight closure of spinal dura mater. Technical note. J. Neurosurg., *43*:639, 1975.
13. Mooney, V.: Innovative approaches to chronic back disability. Instructional course lecture. The American Academy of Orthopaedic Surgeons. Dallas, January, 1974.
14. Nachemson, A. L.: The lumbar spine: An orthopaedic challenge. Spine, *1*:59, 1976.
15. Oudenhover, R. C.: The role of laminectomy, facet rhizotomy and epidural steroids. Spine, *4*:145, 1979.
16. Rose, D. L.: The decompensated back. Arch. Phys. Med. Rehabil., *56*:51, 1975.
17. Rosenthal, J. D., Hahn, J. F., and Martinez, G. J.: A technique for closure of leak of spinal fluid. Surg. Gynecol. Obstet., *140*:948, 1975.
18. Rothman, R. H.: New developments in lumbar disc surgery. Orthop. Rev., *4*:23, 1975.
19. Rothman, R. H., and Simeone, F. A.: The Spine, 2nd ed. Philadelphia, W. B. Saunders Co., 1982.
20. Spengler, D. M., and Freeman, D. W.: Patient selection for lumbar discectomy: An objective approach. Spine, *4*:129, 1979.
21. Tibodeau, A. A.: Management of the problem postoperative back. *In* Proceedings of the American Orthopaedic Association. J. Bone Joint Surg., *55A*:1766, 1973.
22. Waddell, G., Kummell, E. G., Lotto, W. N., Graham, J. D., Hall, H., and McCulloch, J. A.: Failed lumbar disc surgery and repeat surgery following industrial injuries. J. Bone Joint Surg., *61A*:201, 1979.
23. White, A. H., Derby R., and Wynne, G.: Epidural injections for the diagnosis and treatment of low back pain. Spine, *5*:78, 1980.
24. Wilson, J.: Low back pain and sciatica. JAMA, *200*:129, 1967.

Chapter 6

INFECTION

Spinal infection can lead to catastrophic complications for a patient if it is not promptly recognized. However, these infections are only occasionally encountered and treated by most physicians. Nonetheless, they should always be given consideration in the differential diagnosis of spinal lesions and back pain. The goal of this chapter is to review the pertinent anatomy and discuss disc space infections, vertebral osteomyelitis, and tuberculosis of the spine.

ANATOMY

It is generally felt that infections of the spine are secondary to hematogenous spread.[33] The vascular anatomy is similar in the cervical, thoracic, and lumbar areas. Each vertebral body is supplied by multiple small arterial vessels that branch from the major segmental artery. In addition, at each foramen, the posterior spinal artery divides into an ascending and a descending branch. These arteries anastomose with segments above, below, and from the other side to form a network on the posterior surface of each vertebral body. From this complex, three to four nutrient arteries enter the vertebral body through the central foramen.

The venous drainage of the vertebral body is centered posteriorly and is composed of valveless veins.[5] There are three systems that are interconnected: direct veins from the vertebral body; veins between the spinal canal and dura; and external veins. Batson[2] felt that this interconnecting system was responsible for the majority of infections. His observations are especially attractive in explaining the association of urinary tract and pelvic infections with vertebral osteomyelitis. There are proponents of both the arterial system and the venous system as the major source of spinal infections. However, there is no conclusive proof for either explanation. All that can be stated at present is that the theory of infections being blood-borne, either arterial or venous, is certainly plausible. Each route may be involved under certain circumstances.

The blood supply to the intervertebral disc is limited.[4] Small arterial vessels penetrate the disc early in life, but by the third decade, these vascular channels have disappeared. The venous drainage of the intervertebral disc is similar to that of the vertebral body. The probable explanation of primary childhood disc space infections is the vascular supply in the young to the intervertebral disc.

DISC SPACE INFECTIONS

Individuals with primary infections of the disc space can be divided into two groups. One is composed of children, and the other consists of patients who have undergone a previous spine operation. These two entities will be discussed separately.

Disc Space Infections in Children

It is generally accepted that this condition is infectious in nature.[3] The infection is blood-borne through the vascular supply that is present in the intervertebral disc space in children.

When a positive blood culture or biopsy specimen is obtained, *Staphylococcus aureus* is the most frequently found organism. Other organisms that have been found include *Moraxella, Diplococcus*, and diphtheroids. The chance of having a positive blood culture is time-related to the onset of the disease. The earlier the culture is taken, the better the chance for a positive return.[22]

CLINICAL PRESENTATION

Patients can present in a variety of ways. In very young children (under 30 months), the major complaint will be difficulty in walking or standing.[32] The patient usually has a low-grade fever with a history of previous upper respiratory infection. Initially, the hip is the focus of attention, and there is an average delay of 21 days before the correct diagnosis is reached.

The older child may present with abdominal complaints, symptoms caused by meningeal irritation, or back pain. Limitation of back motion, localized tenderness, and hamstring tightness are often elicited. Fever occurs in only about 50 per cent of these patients. Awareness of the possibility of infection along with a careful patient history and physical examination is most important in arriving at a diagnosis.

ROENTGENOGRAPHIC FINDINGS

The upper lumbar spine is the most common area of involvement, although cervical and thoracic infections are reported.[16] The initial x-rays are usually normal, since changes are not detectable for at least three to four weeks after the onset of symptoms. The early roentgenographic changes consist of narrowing of the disc space, irregularity or haziness of the end-plate, and possible cavitation within the end-plate. After one to two months, the end-plate will become sclerotic with partial restoration of the intervertebral space. As the disease progresses, interbody fusion may occur, which can be partial or complete. Finally, multispace involvement can happen, but it is rare, and there is no involvement of the posterior elements. If one is considering infection as a diagnosis but no conventional x-ray changes are found, a bone scan will allow early confirmation.[10]

LABORATORY FINDINGS

The erythrocyte sedimentation rate is the most consistently abnormal finding. The white blood cell count may remain normal or may be only mildly elevated. Blood cultures should always be obtained once the diagnosis of disc space infection comes under consideration. As already mentioned, the earlier these are obtained, the more positive the results. Biopsy is indicated if the physician suspects tuberculosis or if there is a failure to respond to treatment.

TREATMENT

The most important treatment for disc space infection is rest.[6] Some physicians recommend accompanying this recumbency with a body cast. Antistaphylococcal intravenous antibiotics should be initiated after obtaining blood cultures. The treatment should be continued until back pain has disappeared and the sedimentation rate is normal. Surgical intervention is not necessary unless a paravertebral abscess develops.

Postoperative Disc Space Infection

This condition is caused by some type of external violation of the intervertebral disc. In the majority of cases, it follows an operative procedure but has been reported following a needle biopsy, discography, or puncture of a disc during a spinal tap. The incidence following surgery is reported to be between 1 and 3 per cent.[18]

CLINICAL SYMPTOMS AND SIGNS

Anywhere between four to five days to as long as ten weeks following surgery, the patient will complain of severe back pain that may or may not radiate into the legs. There may also be referrral of the pain into the lower abdomen, groin, or testes. The most common physical findings are lumbar muscle spasm and a marked limitation of straight leg raising. The pain complaint is out of proportion to the physical findings. In the majority of patients, there will be no external evidence of infection. The occurrence of temperature elevation is variable and cannot be counted on.

ROENTGENOGRAPHIC CHANGES

Findings on x-ray will follow the onset of symptoms by two to three weeks.[8] The first changes are disc space narrowing along with progressive vertebral end-plate destruction (Fig. 6–1). As the disease process advances, reactive new bone is produced, and this new bone may fill the disc space to result in a spontaneous fusion. Patients who are left with a long fusion appear to function better than those patients without a fusion.[26]

LABORATORY STUDIES

The erythrocyte sedimentation rate is always elevated in this disorder and is the most helpful test. The elevation usually follows the onset of clinical symptoms after several days. A closed needle biopsy of the involved space, though not mandatory, is highly recommended. Although *Staphylococcus aureus* is the most common offending organism,[27] other bacteria can be found, and thus the biopsy will provide microbiologic information for the proper selection of antibacterial agents.

TREATMENT

Bed rest is the principle treatment modality in this type of disc space infection. Some physicians will include plaster immobilization, but this

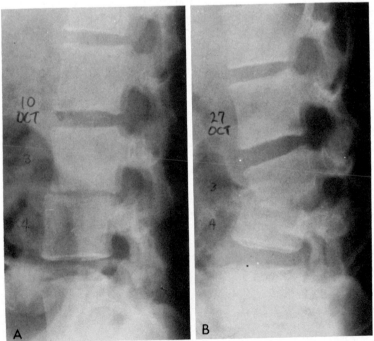

Figure 6–1. *A,* Six weeks postoperative patient presents with low back pain. *B,* Two weeks later there is collapse and destruction at L3–L4 interspace with a proven staphylococcus infection.

treatment is not uniformly applicable. The appropriate antibiotics should be administered, based on the results of a biopsy. Our regimen consists of six weeks of intravenous antibiotics followed by oral drugs until a normal sedimentation rate is reached. The total treatment time usually runs eight to ten weeks. Surgical drainage is necessary only when a paravertebral abscess develops. An abscess should be considered when a patient's pain does not resolve or the sedimentation rate remains elevated despite adequate treatment.

VERTEBRAL OSTEOMYELITIS

Nontubercular vertebral osteomyelitis can lead to serious consequences for the patient. These include paralysis, meningitis, and spinal instability. Thus, it is important to include pyogenic vertebral osteomyelitis in the differential diagnosis of spine lesions. The earlier a spinal infection is diagnosed and treatment is initiated, the better the outcome.

The lumbar spine is the most frequently involved area. In a series reported by Garcia and Grantham,[9] two thirds of the cases involved the lumbar region. However, three quarters of the paravertebral abscesses were found in the cervical and thoracic areas. The fourth lumbar vertebra is most commonly affected; since the introduction of antibiotics, the posterior elements are usually spared.

The aging lumbar spine appears to be more at risk. Eismont and Bohlman, reporting on a series of 65 patients, stated that over 80 per cent of the cases were adults, with an age range from 21 to 80 years.[7] However, the average age was 57, and the median age was 59. These findings highlight the importance of considering the possibility of infection when older patients present with nonmechanical back pain.

ORIGIN OF INFECTION

The source of a spinal infection can be determined in approximately half of the cases.[31] A urinary tract infection is the most common pre-existing focus. The interval between the primary infection and the onset of spine symptoms averages two to three weeks. Other pre-existing infectious sources include the skin, the upper respiratory tract, female genital tract infections, and the bowel in surgery. Drug addiction is increasingly being associated with vertebral osteomyelitis, and iatrogenic infections can occur secondary to closed procedures such as a discogram or needle biopsy.

Staphylococcus aureus is responsible for 90 per cent of adult infections in which positive cultures are obtained. Other possible organisms include *Streptococcus, Escherichia coli, Pseudomonas,* and *Salmonella.* Also, certain clinical presentations are associated with various bacteria. Heroin addicts are prone to infection with gram-negative organisms such as *Pseudomonas* or *E. coli.*[14] Patients with sickle cell disease have a high incidence of *Salmonella* infection.[25]

CLINICAL SIGNS AND SYMPTOMS

The gradual onset of back pain and temperature elevation are the two most consistent complaints. Initially, however, the symptoms and signs may present a highly varied picture as a result of referred pain patterns. Lower thoracic and lumbar involvement may appear as an acute abdomen. In vertebral osteomyelitis secondary to a urinary tract infection, pain and fever may be ascribed to the primary infection. Sciatica may be present if there is nerve root irritation.

On physical examination of the patient, decreased range of motion, muscle spasm, and rigidity are generally present. Distinct percussion tenderness may be noted over the involved spinous processes. In lumbar lesions, when the psoas muscle is irritated, the "hip syndrome" may develop.[23] This syndrome is the complaint of pain with the involved hip held in severe flexion to reduce tension on the psoas muscle.

Different degrees of neurologic loss can be found in these patients. In one reported series of pyogenic vertebral osteomyelitis cases, over 40 per cent had some degree of paralysis. The neurologic deficit can vary from the subjective complaint of sciatica to complete paraplegia. The onset of a progressive neurologic loss may be quite sudden. The treating physician must be aware of this possibility, since immediate surgical intervention is necessary.

Many of these patients will have other significant illnesses. The major associated diseases include diabetes mellitus, chronic alcoholism, various forms of malignancy, and drug addiction. The possibility that there may be a combination of a chronic illness and a developing spinal infection should always be kept in mind.

ROENTGENOGRAPHIC CHANGES

In pyogenic vertebral osteomyelitis, the x-ray changes follow the symptomatic onset of the disease by two to eight weeks[30] (Fig. 6–2). The earliest findings are a narrowing of the disc space, superficial end-plate destruction, and paravertebral soft tissue swelling. As the disease progresses, active destruction of the end-plate and disc space widening are appreciated. Reactive end-plate sclerosis is quite prominent and gives evidence of healing with new bone formation. In many instances, a fusion of the involved vertebral bodies occurs. This can happen between six and 24 months.

These progressive roentgenographic changes must be differentiated from tuberculosis. Unlike pyogenic osteomyelitis, tuberculosis x-ray changes in the spine are usually far advanced by the time symptomatic complaints arise. Also, tuberculosis shows no reactive sclerosis, and fusion takes place from four to six years after the onset of the disease. Other roentgenographic techniques that can be helpful in confirming infection include laminograms to see finer bone detail, technetium bone scans for early diagnosis, and gallium scans to evaluate the paravertebral soft tissues.

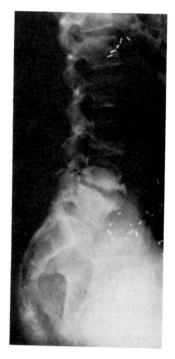

Figure 6–2. Vertebral osteomyelitis with *Staphylococcus epidermidis* in a patient on renal dialysis.

LABORATORY STUDIES

The most consistent abnormal laboratory value is an increased erythrocyte sedimentation rate. The white blood cell count is generally elevated in the young patient (under 20 years of age) but is not a consistent finding in the aging patient.

Bacteriologic verification is strongly recommended; blood cultures should be obtained. Performing a percutaneous needle biopsy is also encouraged. In the lumbar spine, biopsy is a safe technique, and the information received makes the time-consuming procedure worthwhile.

DIAGNOSIS

In any elderly patient who has nonmechanical back pain, the diagnosis of vertebral osteomyelitis has to be considered. An awareness of the possibility of infection is most important. In a series of 65 patients reported by Eismont and Bohlman, the average time from the onset of symptoms to hospitalization was greater than 50 days; once the patient was in the hospital, the average time it took to arrive at a correct diagnosis was greater than 30 days.[7] In this same group, over half of the patients had to be transferred to two or more hospitals before a correct diagnosis was reached. These figures impress the point that the diagnosis of vertebral osteomyelitis can be very elusive. Since these cases have a great potential for serious complications if the diagnosis is not quickly determined and treatment undertaken, every effort should be made to confirm the presence of infection. For this reason, a biopsy is strongly recommended unless existing evidence is unequivocally diagnostic (i.e., routine blood cultures). In many instances, the biopsy will rule out infection but give the correct diagnosis as a metastatic lesion. If one is convinced that an infection is present but all of the diagnostic tests, including needle aspiration, are negative, an open biopsy should be considered. The need for an open biopsy to verify the diagnosis of osteomyelitis is increasing as the variation in the organism (i.e., an increase in gram-negative bacilli) causing vertebral osteomyelitis is seen.[17]

TREATMENT

Immobilization of the spine is the principle treatment of osteomyelitis, and simple bed rest is adequate therapy. However, some physicians advocate the addition of plaster casts or braces. A well-applied plaster jacket will allow a patient to move more comfortably in bed during the initial treatment period. The main indication for using a cast or brace is major bone destruction or instability.

Appropriate antibiotic therapy is also important. Once the correct drug has been chosen by suitable in vitro susceptibility studies, intravenous administration is initiated. It is recommended that patients be treated with parenteral antibiotics for four to six weeks followed by oral antibiotics for a total of six months. The absence of pain and fever and a decrease in the sedimentation rate are the parameters to follow. If the sedimentation rate does not return to normal or the patient's initial presentation demonstrated extensive bony and soft tissue involvement, antibiotics should be continued for a longer period.

Surgical intervention, which includes open biopsy, is indicated when the causative organism is not known, when a paravertebral abscess is present with any sign of spinal cord compression, or with persistent nerve root deficit and lack of response to medical treatment.[15] For pyogenic vertebral osteomyelitis, the anterior approach is strongly recommended. A laminectomy is contraindicated for two reasons: since the spinal cord must be manipulated to gain access to the anterior pathologic feature, the result may be further neurologic loss, and removal of the intact posterior vertebral elements may lead to instability. An anterior approach allows adequate debridement, abscess drainage, and decompression of the spinal cord with bone grafting when indicated.

Paraplegia is a disastrous sequel to vertebral osteomyelitis. There is no clinical means at present to ascertain the degree of irreversible spinal cord damage that is present. Thus, any patient with spinal cord involvement deserves a surgical decompression.

In concluding this section on vertebral osteomyelitis, it should be emphasized that these cases have a tremendous potential for developing serious complications. Awareness of the problem and a carefully considered approach to the diagnosis and treatment are necessary to properly handle these patients.

TUBERCULOSIS OF THE SPINE

The incidence of tuberculosis in the United States has steadily fallen as adequate housing, proper nutrition, and preventive medical measures have become generally available. However, the disease is still quite prevalent in underdeveloped countries. In the United States, there are approximately 31,000 new tuberculosis cases a year, 4000 of which are extrapulmonary.[24] The spine is affected in half of the cases of bone and joint involvement.

Mycobacterium tuberculosis bacilli are strict aerobes, and they will flourish only in areas in which the oxygen tension is high. This is the probable explanation for the vertebral bodies, which are composed mainly of cancellous bone and have a relatively high oxygen tension, becoming involved.[22] There is some controversy over the exact manner in which the bacilli travel to reach the vertebral bodies, although it is generally accepted that it is hematogenous. The most likely route is venous, via Batson's plexus. The first lumbar vertebra is the most commonly affected level, and the incidence of involved segments decreases evenly on either side of L1.

PATHOGENESIS

The pathophysiologic events of tuberculosis are not completely understood. There are two possible states of infection: primary infection, in which bacilli invade a host that has no specific immunity, and adult tuberculosis, in which bacilli produce disease in the case of specific immunity.[24] Adult tuberculosis is often referred to as reinfection, and there is controversy over its pathogenesis. Two possibilities exist: (1) reactivation of foci implanted at the time of the primary infection and (2) reinfection arising from an exogenous source.

Tuberculosis of the spine is always secondary to an active primary focus elsewhere in the body. Once the bacilli reach the vertebral body, metaphysitis, a sequence of granulation tissue with inflammation and caseation necrosis, occurs. If tissue destruction continues, a paraspinal abscess will form. This abscess is composed of necrotic bone and cartilage surrounded by a wall of granulation tissue and edema. The intervertebral disc is usually not involved and lies free within the pus.

The clinical consequences of a paraspinal abscess depend on its size and the anatomic structures it affects. With vertebral body destruction, kyphosis may occur, and if the structural loss is greater on one side than on the other, a component of scoliosis may be founded. If the mechanical integrity of the spinal canal is lost, neural compression will occur, and some degree of paralysis will result. If the abscess is in direct contact with the dura, pachymeningitis may occur.

SIGNS AND SYMPTOMS

Pain is the major complaint of tuberculosis of the spine, and it is aggravated by activity. The pain is centered over the involved area, and the intensity can vary. It can be increased by percussion of the involved vertebrae and on longitudinal compression of the entire vertebral column.

The pain may also be referred to various sites in the body, which will sometimes cause confusion in the diagnosis if this is the initial complaint. The various presentations include simulation of brachialgia, gallbladder disease, or appendicitis. It may also present as girdle pain or buttock and sciatic pain.

Paraplegia or progressive weakness can also be the presenting complaint. Paralysis secondary to tuberculosis was first described by Pott in 1779.[19, 20] In active tuberculosis, paraplegia may result from external pressure on the spinal cord or tuberculi bacilli actually penetrating the dura and involving the spinal cord.

External pressure on the spinal cord is probably the most common etiology of paralysis.[11] The external compression may result from several sources. Pus within an abscess can cause direct pressure. Sequestra or intervertebral discs can exert pressure. Granulation tissue, as it expands, can press upon the spinal cord. Finally, an involved vertebral body can collapse, resulting in a kyphosis with anterior tenting of the spinal cord. When two or more vertebral bodies have been destroyed, instability may occur, with subluxations and dislocations. This is common in the thoracolumbar region, and if the cord is subjected to any pressure, paralysis will result.

Penetration of the dura by the actual tuberculosis infection can occur without paraplegia. However, when the cord is involved, tuberculous meningomyelitis occurs. This is a very grave condition, and the prognosis for any neurologic return is poor.

It should be appreciated that paraplegia may occur after the tuberculosis infection has been successfully treated.[1] This can happen because of transection of the spinal cord by a reactive bony bridge or constriction of the cord by fibrous granulation tissue.

The most common physical finding in the spine is some degree of kyphosis. This is a result of anterior collapse of one or more vertebral bodies. Kyphosis will be most pronounced in the thoracic spine and much less evident in the lumbar spine. With lumbar disease, there will be approximation of the ribs to the iliac crests, with a prominent abdomen.

An abscess may develop with sinus formation. The drainage should always be cultured, for the sinus tract may become secondarily infected. The site of the sinus depends on the level of the disease. An extensive abscess can be present with the patient having no pain and few if any systemic signs of infection. This is commonly referred to as a cold abscess.

X-RAY FINDINGS

X-ray changes are usually far advanced in the spine by the time the disease is clinically appreciated[28] (Fig. 6–3). Paravertebral shadows secondary to edema and abscess formation will be present in the soft tissues. The

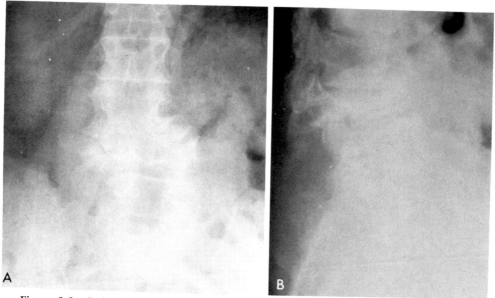

Figure 6–3. Patient with proven tuberculosis of L4. There is significant destruction with collapse.

shadow will vary in shape, depending on the level involved and the size of the abscess. Calcification may be present within the soft tissue shadow.

Bone destruction can be quite significant in tuberculosis. As osteopenia increases within the vertebral bodies, collapse will occur. The various shapes that the destroyed vertebral bodies can take have been described as aneurysmal syndrome, bony bridging, concertina collapses, and reversal of the height-width ratio. If there is a question of spinal cord compression, tomography and myelography may be most helpful.

TREATMENT

The goal in the therapy of tuberculosis is to eradicate the active infection and provide stability for the spine. Three different philosophies exist today in treating spinal tuberculosis. Each of the regimens includes 18 months of chemotherapy. The traditional treatment is nonsurgical, utilizing prolonged bed rest with a plaster jacket.[11] At the other end of the spectrum is the belief that every vertebral lesion should be surgically treated.[11] Our feeling is that a "middle-path" regimen should be followed, as advocated by Tuli[29] in India and Riska[21] in Finland.

Rest and chemotherapy are the initial treatment modalities. Rest is enforced, and a plaster jacket is used, if necessary. Once the diagnosis is made, drugs are administered. The exact chemotherapy regimen can vary from institution to institution, and it is suggested that an infectious disease consultation be obtained to direct drug therapy. The patients are followed on a periodic basis (usually every three months) with radiographs and determinations of erythrocyte sedimentation rates. Progressive ambulation is started at six to nine months if the pain has disappeared, the sedimentation rate is reduced, and the x-ray is satisfactory. A spinal orthosis will be most helpful to the patient in the initial stages of mobilization.

Surgical intervention is recommended for patients who do not respond to chemotherapy and rest. The failure is denoted by continued pain with at least three months of treatment and an increasing sedimentation rate. Patients who present with a neurologic loss and fail to respond to conservative therapy or patients who develop paraplegia while under adequate treatment are definite surgical candidates. Patients who have an unstable spine (progressive kyphosis) or a paravertebral abscess need surgical treatment. Abscesses, however, may be superficial and palpable, in which case aspiration and instillation of antibiotics have proved to be most successful. If the abscess is deep or does not respond to antibiotics, surgery is necessary. Finally, in a few instances, surgery is needed to confirm the diagnosis.

The goal of surgery is to remove all of the infected tissue, which can include pus, sequestrated intervertebral discs, bony sequestra, and granulation tissue. The second aim of a procedure is to leave the patient with a stable spine. This is best accomplished by a fusion. Since the infection is usually anterior, an anterior approach is recommended.[13] This will allow the surgeon, under excellent exposure, to eradicate the infection, decompress the neural elements, and perform a solid fusion.

REFERENCES

1. Bailey, H. L., Gabriel, M., Hodgson, A. R., and Shin, J. S.: Tuberculosis of the spine. J. Bone Joint Surg., *54A*:1633, 1972.
2. Batson, O. V.: The vertebral vein system: Caldwell lecture, 1956. Am. J. Roentgenol. Radium Ther. Nucl. Med., *78*:195, 1957.
3. Boston, H. C., Bianco, A. J., and Rhodes, K. H.: Disc space infections in children. Orthop. Clin. North Am., *6*:953, 1975.
4. Coventry, M. B., Ghormley, R. K., and Kernohan, J. W.: The intervertebral disc: its microscopic anatomy and pathology. Part I. Anatomy, development, and physiology. J. Bone Joint Surg., *27*:105, 1945.
5. Crock, H. V., Yoshizawa, H., and Kame, S. K.: Observations on the venous drainage of the human vertebral body. J. Bone Joint Surg., *55B*:528, 1973.
6. Dich, V. Q., Nelson, J. D., and Haltalin, K. C.: Osteomyelitis in infants and children — a review of 163 cases. Am. J. Dis. Child., *129*:1273, 1975.
7. Eismont, F. J., and Bohlman, H. H.: Pyogenic and fungal vertebral osteomyelitis — a review of sixty-five cases. Read at the Annual Meeting of the AAOS, Las Vegas, Nevada, 1977.
8. Ford, L. T., and Key, J. A.: Postoperative infection of interbertebral disc space. South. Med. J., *48*:1295, 1955.
9. Garcia, A., and Grantham, A.: Hematogenous pyogenic vertebral osteomyelitis. J. Bone Joint Surg., *42A*:429, 1960.
10. Gelfand, M. J., and Silberstein, E. E.: Radionuclide imaging — use in diagnosis of osteomyelitis in children. JAMA, *237*:245, 1977.
11. Griffith, D. L. L, Seddon, H. J., and Roaf, R.: Pott's Paraplegia. London, Oxford University Press, 1956.
12. Hodgson, A. R., Skinsnes, O. K., and Leong, C. Y.: The pathogenesis of Pott's paraplegia. J. Bone Joint Surg., *49A*:1147, 1967.
13. Hodgson, A. R., and Stock, F. E.: Anterior spine fusion for the treatment of tuberculosis of the spine. J. Bone Joint Surg., *42A*:295, 1960.
14. Holzman, R. S., and Bishko, F.: Osteomyelitis in heroin addicts. Ann. Intern. Med., *75*:693, 1971.
15. Kemp, H. B. S., Jackson, J. W., Jeremiah, J. D., and Cook, J.: Anterior fusion of the spine for infective lesions in adults. J. Bone Joint Surg., *55B*:715, 1973.

16. Milone, F. P., Bianco, A. J., Jr., and Ivins, J. C.: Infections of the intervertebral disc in children. JAMA, *181*:1029, 1962.
17. Nagel, D. A., Albright, J. A., Keggi, K. H., and Southwick, W. O.: Closer look at spinal lesions: open biopsy of vertebral lesions. JAMA, *191*:975, 1965.
18. Pilgaard, S.: Discitis (closed space infection) following removal of lumbar intervertebral disc. J. Bone Joint Surg. (Am), *51*:713, 1969.
19. Pott, P.: Remarks on that Kind of Palsy of the Lower Limbs Which is Frequently Found to Accompany a Curvature of the Spine and is Supposed to be Caused by it, Together with its Method of Cure. London, 1779.
20. Pott, P.: Further Remarks on the Useless State of the Lower Limbs in Consequence of a Curvature of the Spine. London, 1782.
21. Riska, E. B.: Spinal tuberculosis treated by antituberculous chemotherapy and radical operation. Clin. Orthop., *119*:148, 1976.
22. Rocco, H. D., and Eyring, E. J.: Intervertebral disc infections in children. Am. J. Dis. Child., *123*:448, 1972.
23. Ross, P. M., and Fleming, J. L.: Vertebral body osteomyelitis — spectrum and natural history — a retrospective analysis of 37 cases. Clin. Orthop., *118*:190, 1976.
24. Rothman, R. H., and Simeone, F.: The Spine. Philadelphia, W. B. Saunders Co., 1982.
25. Schweitzer, G., Hoosen, G. M., and Dunbar, J. M.: Salmonella typhi spondylitis: an unusual presentation. S. Afr. Med. J., *45*:126, 1971.
26. Sullivan, C. R., Bickel, W. H., and Svien, H. J.: Infections of vertebral interspaces after operations on intervertebral disks. JAMA, *166*:1973, 1958.
27. Thibodeau, A. A.: Closed space infection following removal of lumbar intervertebral disc. J Bone Joint Surg. (Am), *50*:400, 1968.
28. Tuli, S. M., Srivastava, T. P., Varma, B. P., and Sinha, G. P.: Tuberculosis of spine. Acta Orthop. Scand., *38*:445, 1967.
29. Tuli, S. M.: Results of treatment of spina tuberculosis by "middle-path" regime. J Bone Joint Surg., *57B*:13, 1975.
30. Waldvogel, F. A., Medoff, G., and Swartz, M. N.: Osteomyelitis: a review of clinical features, therapeutic considerations and unusual aspects. N. Engl. J. Med., *28*:316, 1970.
31. Waldvogel, F. A., and Vasey, H.: Osteomyelitis: the past decade. N. Engl. J. Med., *303*:360, 1980.
32. Wenger, D. R., Bobechko, W. P., Cilday, D. L.: The spectrum of intervertebral disc-space infection in children. J. Bone Joint Surg., *60A*:100, 1978.
33. Wiley, A. M., Truetta, J.: The vascular anatomy of the spine and its relationship to pyogenic vertebral osteomyelitis. J. Bone Joint Surg., *41B*:796, 1959.

Chapter 7

TUMORS

Tumors involving the lumbar spine are a relatively uncommon occurrence. However, the consequences of a neoplastic spine lesion are so disastrous that the physician should keep the possibility of its existence in mind when dealing with back pain of unclear etiology. The purpose of this section is to review the neoplastic diseases more commonly found in the aging lumbar spine. These will include metastatic disease, multiple myeloma, chondrosarcoma, hemangioma, and chordoma.

METASTATIC DISEASE

Seventy per cent of primary malignant tumors will be found to have metastasized to bone if autopsies are performed.[2] The spine is the most commonly involved site. Approximately 60 per cent of metastatic carcinomas found in bone are in the spine. The lumbar region of the spine is the most common area affected, although metastatic disease has been reported at every level of the spinal column.

The most common primary tumor to spread to the spine is prostatic carcinoma in the male and breast carcinoma in the female.[20] However, any malignant neoplasm may metastasize to the spine. Other frequently found metastatic tumors arise from the gastrointestinal tract, kidneys, thyroid, and lungs.

The early diagnosis of metastatic spine disease is dependent on the treating physician having a high index of suspicion. In patients over the age of 40 who have low back pain of questionable etiology, the possibility of a tumor should always be considered.

The patient's history is not specific. Pain is the major presenting complaint. Many times the patient will state that the pain is worse at night and is not exacerbated by periods of activity. Unfortunately, this pain history does not always hold true for metastatic disease.[13] Non-neoplastic disease of the spine can also present in this fashion. When the neurologic elements are involved, the patient may complain of urinary, bowel, or sexual dysfunction.[12] The physician must specifically ask about not only these problems but also about a prior history of a neoplastic process. In general, if a patient gives a history of having had a tumor, it must be assumed until proven otherwise that the current problems are connected with it.

150

The physical examination is also not specific for reaching a diagnosis. Local tenderness, muscle spasm, and limited motion may be present. If the metastatic lesion has caused a neurologic deficit, the physical examination may help in localizing the anatomic area involved. However, a positive neurologic exam only means that there is compression of the nerve roots or spinal cord and that the etiology will need further definition.

ROENTGENOGRAPHIC APPEARANCE

Routine roentgenographic examination will demonstrate an alteration in the architecture of the bone. The neoplastic lesions are generally found in the vertebral body within the spine.[29] These metastatic lesions have classically been described as osteolytic or osteoblastic. The vast majority of lesions are osteolytic or destructive in their effect (Fig. 7–1). The main osteoblastic lesion arises from prostatic carcinoma. It should be appreciated that breast tumors, which usually produce osteolytic lesions in the spine, can also lead to osteoblastic changes. In fact, one can see both osteoblastic and osteolytic lesions secondary to breast cancer in the same patient.[18]

In many instances, the plain x-ray examination will be normal, but the clinical picture for a particular patient will still cause suspicion of a neoplastic process as the underlying problem. In this situation, a technetium bone scan is the most effective diagnostic test to survey not only the spine but the entire skeleton for a "hidden" malignancy.[8] In fact, in any elderly patient who has continuous low back pain that does not respond to treatment, a bone scan is performed to rule out an occult tumor. Also, a

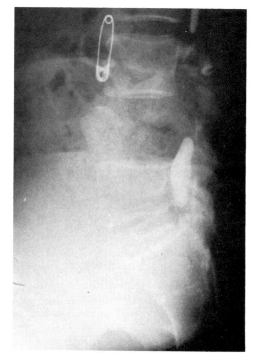

Figure 7–1. Fifty-four year old female presenting with back and right leg pain. Patient was found to have breast carcinoma with an osteolytic lesion to L4.

metastatic lesion can be superimposed on another pathologic process. The most common pathologic processes in the spine are degenerative disease and osteoporosis. Thus, a bone scan is ordered if an older patient with a known spinal problem experiences a change in symptoms.

LABORATORY FINDINGS

Laboratory studies can be most helpful in diagnosing cancer. Once the possibility of an underlying malignancy has arisen, there are several blood studies that should be routinely performed. These include a complete blood count, sedimentation rate, urinalysis, and the levels of calcium, phosphorus, alkaline phosphatase, and acid phosphatase (in the male). If the situation warrants it, more complex studies are obtained, such as a protein electrophoresis to rule in or rule out specific entities, such as multiple myeloma.

There are several clinical situations that may arise in metastatic disease. The most common is the patient with a known primary cancer who develops back pain and subsequently is found to have a lesion in the spine. The other major clinical setting is the patient who has *no* known primary cancer and who develops a destructive spinal process. In the latter case, the etiology of the lesion must be established. Other causes for the destructive process, such as metabolic disease or infection, have to be ruled out. A specimen of spinal tissue is usually needed to determine an accurate diagnosis. In the lumbar spine, this is relatively easy to accomplish using a closed needle biopsy. Although it is time-consuming, a needle biopsy will yield high returns if correctly and carefully performed.[9] Occasionally, in spite of the best technique, the biopsy specimen will be reported as normal or read as metastatic cancer, primary source unknown. At this point, a "metastatic work-up" is initiated and proceeds until the primary tumor is uncovered.

TREATMENT

The therapy employed in metastatic lumbar spine cancer is oriented toward palliation of the pain, which may be intractable. The pain originates from the metastatic lesion itself or is secondary to a compression fracture if the destruction is great enough.[4] Radiotherapy is the mainstay of treatment.[3] The type of machine and dose of radiotherapy vary widely according to the institution. If there is no neurologic involvement, dramatic pain relief can be achieved, although the amount of pain relief is unpredictable in an individual patient. Metastatic lesions from the breast, lung, and thyroid are the most sensitive to radiotherapy.

Neurologic loss is a disastrous consequence of metastatic spine lesions. Involvement of the thoracic area leads to the highest incidence of paralysis, but it can occur in the lumbar spine as well.[16] Once paraplegia has occurred secondary to a metastatic lesion in the lumbar spine, surgical intervention will not lead to any functional return. However, a laminectomy is recommended in cases of incomplete paraplegia.[30] The major goal in this instance is to prevent further progression of paralysis, although mild neurologic improvement has been reported. Once a neurologic deficit has been noted, the faster that surgery is undertaken, the better the results.

MULTIPLE MYELOMA

Multiple myeloma is a distinctive malignant neoplasm that originates from hematopoietic cells in the bone marrow.[14] It is the most common primary tumor of bone. Myeloma can clinically present as a localized osseous lesion or, as the name implies, affect multiple sites as a systemic disease. It is most often discovered in patients between the ages of 40 and 60, and males are more commonly affected than females.

The etiology of multiple myeloma is unclear.[24] It is associated with a proliferation of plasma cells in the bone marrow, and there are some who feel that it is not a true cancer but rather an abnormality in the blood-forming apparatus. Regardless of its origin, the disease presents definite clinicoanatomic features that sharply define it from other blood-related tumors.

Pain is the most commonly presenting complaint in multiple myeloma. Initially, the pain is often vague and is associated with a feeling of weakness. The vertebral body is the most commonly involved bone, and thus, unexplained back pain in the elderly should alert the physician to the possibility of myeloma.[6] Frequently, a single vertebral body will collapse and a compression fracture will be the presenting picture. This can be associated with mild trauma. Depending on the degrees of vertebral destruction, compression of the spinal cord or nerve roots can occur.[11] This neural compression may be progressive and is usually associated with intense pain. The other common finding is weight loss.

LABORATORY FINDINGS

The increase in plasma cells in multiple myeloma results in a variety of abnormal laboratory studies. The major finding is the appearance of a distinctive immunoglobulin that may be found in both the urine and the blood.[26] In the urine, it is commonly referred to as the Bence Jones protein and is strongly suggestive of the disease. However, the absence of this protein does not rule out myeloma, for it occurs in only about half of the cases. The protein is discovered by performing a protein electrophoresis on either the blood or the urine.

Anemia is also a commonly associated finding in plasma cell myeloma. This is probably secondary to the invasion of the marrow by plasma cells. The complaint of fatigue coupled with an unexplained anemia in an older patient should alert the physician. Other abnormal blood studies include an increased sedimentation rate, a reversal of the normal albumin/globulin ratio, and an increase in the serum alkaline phosphatase and serum calcium levels.

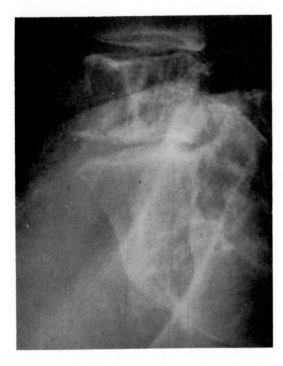

Figure 7–2. Sixty-eight year old male with unremitting low back pain. Myeloma was eventual diagnosis. X-ray demonstrates lytic lesion of L5. (From Rothman, R. H., and Simeone, F. A.: The Spine, 1st ed. Philadelphia, W. B. Saunders Co., 1975.)

A conclusive diagnosis is reached by performing a biopsy on a suspected lesion.[31] The area of bone involvement may be technically difficult to reach, and in many instances, a bone marrow puncture from either the sternum or the iliac crest will substitute. The histologic picture from either the involved site or a marrow aspirate will demonstrate an increased number of both typical and atypical plasma cells.

Roentgenographic Appearance

The characteristic appearance of a multiple myeloma lesion is a radiolucent deficit without any significant new bone formation[15] (Fig. 7–2). There is no reactive sclerosis, and the lesions are sharply demarcated. Any bone can be affected, and as already mentioned, the vertebral bodies are the most common bones involved. In many instances, the initial complaint is the onset of acute back pain associated with mild trauma. An x-ray will detect an isolated compression fracture with normal adjacent vertebral bodies. This presentation should make the physician suspicious of a destructive process with a secondary fracture. The most common underlying process is either metastatic carcinoma or multiple myeloma. Further diagnostic studies may include a bone marrow puncture or a biopsy of the lesion, which will generally lead to the correct diagnosis.

Treatment

Currently, there is no curative therapy available for multiple myeloma.[1] Systemic multiple drug chemotherapy is being employed with prolonged survival times. Radiation is instituted for a locally painful lesion, which is relatively common in the spine. Surgery of the spine is contemplated only when there is instability or a progressive loss of neurologic function. These cases are difficult, and each requires individual planning.

CHONDROSARCOMA

Chondrosarcoma is the most common primary malignant neoplasm (excluding multiple myeloma) that occurs in the lumbar spine.[17] Its overall incidence in the spine is estimated to be 6 per cent. The disease is most prevalent in patients over the age of 40, and males have a higher incidence than females.

Chondrosarcoma can be defined as a malignant cartilaginous neoplasm.[25] It may develop de novo in bone or arise from pre-existing cartilaginous tissue. The former are referred to as primary lesions, whereas the latter are regarded as secondary chondrosarcomas. Only in the relatively recent past has chondrosarcoma been separated into a distinct entity from osteogenic sarcoma. This separation is most important, for the prognosis is quite different in the two tumors. Chondrosarcoma grows at a much slower rate than osteogenic sarcoma and, consequently, metastasizes much later in its course. Thus, aggressive surgical treatment of chondrosarcoma at an early stage can provide a much better prognosis than can osteogenic sarcoma.

Clinically, pain is the most common presenting symptom. Occasionally, when the spine is involved, a neurologic loss may be associated with the pain. Depending on the location of the tumor, the neurologic deficit may

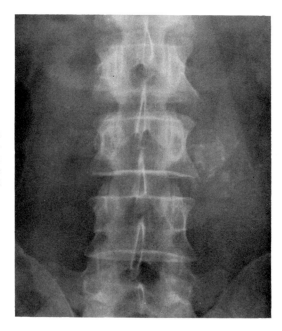

Figure 7–3. Transverse process of third lumbar vertebra demonstrates chondrosarcoma. Radio-dense regions are present. (From Rothman, R. H., and Simeone, F. A.: The Spine, 1st ed. Philadelphia, W. B. Saunders Co., 1975.)

consist of root irritation or a progressive significant neurologic loss. In the sacral area, a chondrosarcoma may initially present with a disturbance of bowel, bladder, or sexual dysfunction.

Roentgenographic appearance

Radiologically, chondrosarcomas display an osteolytic central area with radiodense regions[5] (Fig. 7–3). The basic tumor is destructive and is responsible for the lytic area. The radiodense areas represent spotty calcification and ossification of the neoplasm. In many cases, the calcification will be so thick that the individual lobules are outlined. Computerized axial tomography is helpful in these spinal lesions to evaluate the degree of canal involvement and the amount of soft tissue that is affected.

The diagnosis of chondrosarcoma necessitates a biopsy with histologic evaluation.[22] At the present time, there are no specific laboratory tests for diagnosis. Both the anterior and posterior elements may be involved in the spine, and the tumor can extend from one level to another.

Treatment

Treatment is directed at surgical removal of the tumor mass. In the spine, it is rare that a complete excision can be accomplished, but because of a chondrosarcoma's slow growth, resection of as much tumor as possible is beneficial. Some patients can be kept alive for many years by repeated excisions of the tumor mass.[21] If there is neurologic compromise, the surgical goal should be relief of the mechanical pressure. The physician should consider stabilization from the beginning, since tumor resection may lead to instability. Radiation and chemotherapy are not effective in chondrosarcoma because of the slow-growing nature of the neoplasm.

CHORDOMA

Chordoma is a tumor that originates from remaining notochordal tissue.[10] It is a rare neoplasm. However, over 90 per cent of the reported cases occur in the upper or lower end of the vertebral column, with the sacrococcygeal and lumbar regions being the most commonly involved. It is a disease of the older population. Most patients are over the age of 50, and males are affected twice as often as females.

Chordomas are very slow-growing neoplasms and may be present for many years before they cause significant complaints. Symptoms result from either invasion or pressure. Metastases are reported in less than 10 per cent of patients and may involve the lungs, bone, soft tissue, or liver.[32] Metastases spread via the lymphatic system and usually occur in patients with long-standing disease.

Pain is the initial complaint of chordoma. In many instances, it is of long duration and progressive in nature. Occasionally, patients will present with constipation as a result of direct rectal pressure or urologic and neurologic signs secondary to tumor invasion.

The physical examination can be very rewarding. If the tumor mass is anterior on the sacrum, the rectum can be pushed further forward into the pelvis. In this case, a rectal examination will reveal a firm or semicystic mass on the posterior wall of the rectum. Localizing neurologic findings may also be present if the tumor has spread and invaded the surrounding neural elements.

ROENTGENOGRAPHIC APPEARANCE

The roentgenographic picture of a chordoma is one of lysis (Fig. 7–4). In the sacral area, there may be a large lytic lesion in the midline that is usually associated with a presacral soft tissue mass.[19] There may also be calcification within the tumor border. If the neoplasm is in the lumbar spine, vertebral body destruction is noted because the notochordal remnants exist within the center of the vertebral bodies. To delineate the size of the tumor and the structures that are involved, computer axial tomography is most helpful. In trying to establish an early diagnosis, a bone scan is useful. However, it is not specific for chordoma.

The diagnosis of chordoma is dependent on obtaining a piece of tissue for histologic study, which will demonstrate a loose mucinous matrix with physaliphorous cells.[7] An open biopsy may not be an innocuous procedure, owing to the tumor location. When possible, a needle aspiration biopsy

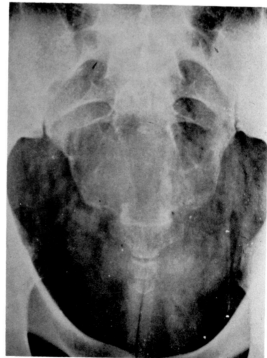

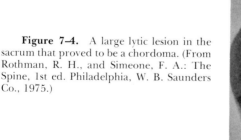

Figure 7–4. A large lytic lesion in the sacrum that proved to be a chordoma. (From Rothman, R. H., and Simeone, F. A.: The Spine, 1st ed. Philadelphia, W. B. Saunders Co., 1975.)

should be performed to obtain tissue. This is usually possible in the lumbar spine but not in the sacrococcygeal region.

TREATMENT

To date, the treatment of chordomas has proven somewhat disappointing. Surgical ablation is difficult, and hemicorporectomy for sacrococcygeal lesions seems unwise in the majority of cases. Because of the tumor's slow growth, periodic debulking procedures may increase survival time, prevent or delay neurologic involvement, or both. High voltage radiation treatment can be used for palliation, but chordomas are not radiosensitive and the results are poor.

HEMANGIOMA

Hemangioma is a soft tissue tumor found in bone.[27] It is composed of vascular channels and may be either capillary or cavernous in nature. Capillary hemangiomas are composed of large spaces between normal bone trabeculae. The cavernous type reveals dense fibrous tissue with vascular channels scattered throughout. In the spine, symptomatic hemangiomas are relatively rare. However, necropsy studies by Fopfer and others have determined the overall incidence to be 12 per cent.[23] The incidence increases with age, affecting 4.5 per cent of people under 20 years old as compared with 36 per cent of people over 50 years of age. Symptomatic hemangiomas are most commonly seen in the 30- to 50-year-old group, with males and females equally represented. Though it may affect any bone, the spine is the most frequent site of hemangiomas, and it is not unusual for two or more contiguous bodies to be involved.

Pain and tenderness over the involved vertebrae are the usual presenting symptoms. Because of the tumor's insidious nature, pain may be of long duration before a physician is consulted. Infrequently, in the lumbar spine, a patient may present with a neurologic deficit secondary to compression of the cauda equina. Hemangiomas can cause this compression by expansion of an involved vertebra, resulting in a narrowing of the spinal canal, direct extension of the tumor into the extradural space, compression fracture of an involved vertebra, or extradural hematoma secondary to the neoplasm.

ROENTGENOGRAPHIC APPEARANCE

The usual roentgenographic picture of a hemangioma in the spine is prominent vertical striations in the vertebral body with near absence of the horizontal trabeculae owing to their absorption[28] (Fig. 7–5). The entire vertebral body is affected with little change in its overall shape. This x-ray presentation is classic for hemangioma and makes the diagnosis relatively easy. Unfortunately, hemangiomas may demonstrate atypical x-ray fea-

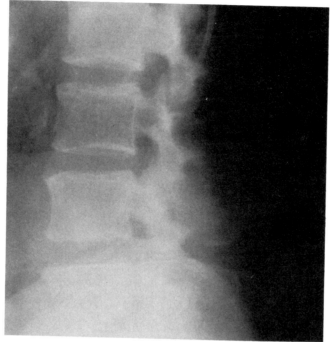

Figure 7–5. Hemangioma of L3 demonstrating prominent vertical striations.

tures, such as pedicular erosion, paravertebral soft tissue masses, or bony expansion. This can make the diagnosis difficult, and in the older age group, the physician will usually have to differentiate metastatic disease from hemangioma.

TREATMENT

The principal treatment of hemangiomas is irradiation. This should be instituted as soon as the diagnosis is made to prevent any neural compression. If the patient presents with a neural deficit, surgical decompression is indicated. Technically, decompression can be quite difficult because of excessive bleeding. Therefore, it is recommended that a preoperative spinal angiogram be performed to delineate the blood supply to the tumor. This will allow the surgeon to safely ligate the blood supply to the tumor while avoiding the anterior spinal artery. It should be appreciated that irradiation therapy is most successful in affecting relief of symptoms in the majority of cases and that surgery is only rarely indicated.

REFERENCES

1. Alexanian, R., Salmon, S., Bonnet, J., Gehan, E., Haut, A., and Weick, J.: Combination therapy for multiple myeloma. Cancer, *40*:2765, 1977.
2. American Cancer Society: 1970 Cancer Facts and Figures. The American Cancer Society, Inc., 1969.

3. Bansal, S., et al.: The treatment of metastatic spinal cord tumors. JAMA, *202*:126, 1967.

4. Bhalla, S. K.: Metastatic disease of the spine. Clin. Orthop., *73*:52, 1970.

5. Barnes, R., and Catto, M.: Chondrosarcoma of bone. J. Bone Joint Surg., *48B*:729, 1966.

6. Carson, C. P., Ackerman, L. V., and Maltby, J. D.: Plasma cell myeloma. A clinical, pathologic, and roentgenologic review of 90 cases. Am. J. Clin. Pathol., *25*:849, 1955.

7. Congdon, C. C.: Benign and malignant chordomas. A clinico-anatomical study of twenty-two cases. Am. J. Pathol., *28*:793, 1952.

8. Craig, F. S.: Metastatic and primary lesions of bone. Clin. Orthop., *73*:33, 1970.

9. Craig, F. S.: Vertebral body biopsy. J. Bone Joint Surg., *38A*:93, 1956.

10. Dahlin, D. C., and MacCarty, C. S.: Chordoma. A study of 59 cases. Cancer, *5*:1170, 1952.

11. Davison, C., and Balser, B. H.: Myeloma and its neural complications. Arch. Surg., *35*:913, 1937.

12. Fager, C. A.: Management of malignant intraspinal disease. Surg. Clin. North Am., *47*:743, 1967.

13. Francis, K. C., and Hutter, V. P.: Neoplasms of the spine in the aged. Clin. Orthop., *26*:54, 1963.

14. Gorji, J., and Francis, K. C.: Multiple myeloma. Clin. Orthop., *38*:106, 1965.

15. Gross, R. E., and Vaughan, W. W.: Plasma cell myeloma. Am. J. Roentgenol., *39*:344, 1938.

16. Hardy, H. I. M., and Dugger, C. S.: Myelopathy caused by metastatic spinal epidural neoplasms. South. Med. J., *60*:72, 1967.

17. Henderson, E. D., and Dahlin, D. C.: Chondrosarcoma of bone. A study of 288 cases. J. Bone Joint Surg., *45A*:1450, 1963.

18. Henson, R. A., Russell, D. S., and Wilkinson, M.: Carcinomatous neuropathy and myopathy. A clinical and pathological study. Brain, 77:82, 1954.

19. Higginbotham, N. L., Phillips, R. F., Farr, H. W., and Husto, H. O.: Chordoma. Thirty-five year study at Memorial Hospital. Cancer, *20*:1841, 1967.

20. Jaffe, H. L.: Tumors and tumorous conditions of the bones and joints. Philadelphia, Lea and Febiger, 1958.

21. Lichtenstein, L.: Diseases of bone and joints. St. Louis, C. V. Mosby Co., 1970.

22. Lichtenstein, L., and Jaffee, H. L.: Chondrosarcoma of bone. Am. J. Pathol., *19*:553, 1943.

23. Marcial-Rojas, R. A.: Primary hemangiopericytoma of bone. Review of the literature and report of the first case with metastases. Cancer, *13*:308, 1960.

24. Meyer, J. E., and Schulz, M. D.: "Solitary" myeloma of bone. Cancer, *34*:438, 1974.

25. O'Neal, L. W., and Ackerman, L. V.: Chondrosarcoma of bone. Cancer, *5*:551, 1952.

26. Osserman, E. F., and Lawlor, D. P.: Abnormal serum and urine proteins in 35 cases of multiple myeloma, as studied by filter paper electrophoresis. Am. J. Med., *18*:462, 1955.

27. Otis, J., Hutter, R. V. P., Foote, F. W., Jr., Marcove, R. C., and Stewart, F. W.: Hemangioendothelioma of bone. Surg. Gynecol. Obstet., *127*:295, 1968.

28. Sherman, R. S., and Wilner, D.: The roentgen diagnosis of hemangioma of bone. Am. J. Roentgenol., *86*:1146, 1961.

29. Turner, J. W., and Jaffe, H. L.: Metastatic neoplasms. Am. J. Roentgenol., *43*:479, 1940.

30. Vieth, R. G., and Odom, G. L.: Extradural spinal metastases and their neurosurgical treatment. J. Neurosurg., *23*:501, 1965.

31. Waldenstrom, J.: Diagnosis and treatment of multiple myeloma. New York, Grune and Stratton, Inc., 1970.

32. Wang, C. C., and James, A. E.: Chordoma: brief review of the literature and report of a case with widespread metastases. Cancer, *22*:162, 1968.

Chapter 8

METABOLIC BONE DISEASE AS PRESENTED BY THE SPINE

The term "metabolic bone disease" infers that multiple osseous structures throughout the body are affected. In many instances, the disease entity initially presents as back pain. This is particularly true in the older patient. Thus, it is important for the spinal surgeon to include metabolic bone disease in the differential diagnosis of back pain in the elderly patient. In other words, awareness of the problem is the initial step toward identifying the disease process. The goal of this chapter is to present an organized approach to use for the patient with a potential metabolic bone disease and to review some of the major metabolic disorders that may initially present as a spinal problem. These include osteoporosis, osteomalacia, hyperparathyroidism, Paget's disease, and gout. The choice of the diseases that are discussed is somewhat arbitrary. However, they can all present as back discomfort in the aging patient, affect bones other than the spine, and cause symptoms on a nonmechanical basis. It should be emphasized that this chapter is not a comprehensive coverage of the various diseases but rather an overview, with specific attention directed toward lumbar spine involvement in the aging patient.

PATIENT EVALUATION

History

There is no specific symptom complex of the back associated with the metabolic bone diseases. Pain is the primary presenting complaint, and it does not usually have a mechanical basis. However, with compression fractures of the vertebral bodies secondary to a metabolic disturbance, the pain may have a mechanical character. Other symptoms include muscular weakness, inability to walk stairs, and vague localized pains, especially in the peripheral joints.[16] The important point is that all of the older population has the potential of having a metabolic bone disease. If the investigating physician cannot find a specific diagnosis to account for a patient's complaint, he should consider a metabolic etiology and proceed with the appropriate work-up.

PHYSICAL EXAMINATION

Kyphoscoliosis is the most common physical finding in the metabolic bone diseases.[4] This may be a progressive problem in osteopenic conditions and may be associated with vertebral body compression fractures. There is usually no neurologic involvement, and thus the neurologic examination and tension signs are routinely found to be within normal limits. A paucity of objective findings in combination with nonspecific subjective complaints should alert the examining physician to an underlying metabolic disturbance.

DIAGNOSTIC STUDIES

Once the suspicion of a metabolic abnormality has arisen, there are a number of diagnostic tests that are helpful. Some of the studies are useful in ruling out other entities, such as tumor or infection, that are high on the differential list when a diagnosis of metabolic bone disease is being considered. The degree of sophistication of these studies ranges from very simple to most difficult, and in general, the more difficult it is to perform these tests, the harder they are to interpret and the less helpful they are in the everyday clinical setting. Therefore, it is beneficial to develop an organized progression of diagnostic studies for patients with possible metabolic bone disease. A haphazard approach is usually unsuccessful and can be very frustrating for both the physician and the patient. The general outline and temporal progression of the tests we employ are depicted in Table 8–1.[28] The interpretation of each of these studies will be discussed along with the appropriate clinical entity.

OSTEOPOROSIS

Osteoporosis is the loss of absolute bone mass with the ratio of the bone's mineral content compared with its osteoid content remaining normal.[34] This loss of bone mass can be termed osteopenia and predominantly affects the trabecular bone of the spinal column, femoral necks, and the ends of long bones.

TABLE 8–1. Diagnostic Studies in Metabolic Bone Disease

Stage I	CBC, sedimentation rate, BUN, creatinine, uric acid, Ca/PO$_4$, alkaline phosphatase, acid phosphatase, Rh factor, HLA-B-27, ANA Plain x-rays Urinalysis
Stage II	Bone scan, parathyroid hormone assay, T-3 level, corticol level, protein electrophoresis
Stage III	Bone biopsy (iliac crest)
Stage IV	GI absorption tests

PATHOPHYSIOLOGY

Absolute bone loss is the result of bone resorption in excess of bone formation.[17] Normally, bone resorption increases with age. An individual normally begins to lose bone at the age of 40. In general, males have more bone mass than females, and blacks have more bone mass than whites. Males usually lose between 5 and 8 per cent of their bone mass every decade, whereas females lose between 10 and 15 per cent of their bone mass every ten years.[32] Osteoporotic patients are individuals whose bone loss exceeds the just-mentioned figures. One third of white women will develop clinically significant osteoporosis.

The actual cause of osteoporosis is unknown. It is likely that several mechanisms are involved. Mewnier estimates that 10 per cent of osteoporotic patients have excessive osteoclastic activity resulting in a rapid turnover state, 30 per cent have defective osteoblastic function resulting in a slow turnover state, and the remaining 60 per cent have normal turnover skeletal states with some type of imbalance between the rates of bone formation and resorption.[1] This infers that there is a defective "coupling" of the cellular processes involved in bone resorption and formation. Exactly what this defect consists of is presently unknown. Once the other metabolic causes of osteopenia (osteomalacia and endocrine abnormalities) have been ruled out, the physician is left with an unknown absolute bone mass loss. In the past, adult osteoporosis consisted of three subdivisions: idiopathic, found in men under 50, postmenopausal, and senile. However, there has been a continuous increase in the appearance of osteoporosis in persons from age 40 until senility in both sexes.[9] Thus, the above three groups are now termed primary osteoporosis. Primary osteoporosis does not include juvenile osteoporosis or bone loss caused by known endocrine or metabolic abnormalities.

CLINICAL SIGNS AND SYMPTOMS

Postmenopausal white females are the most commonly affected group. Fortunately, the course of the disease is benign in the majority of patients (95 per cent). In about 3 per cent of patients between 40 and 60 years of age, osteoporosis is progressive, severely disabling, and an impediment to the activities of everyday living.[33] Back pain secondary to multiple vertebral body compression fractures is the most frequent picture. These compression fractures are in many instances associated with a progressively increasing kyphoscoliosis. This disabling deformity is commonly referred to as the "dowager's hump." As the kyphoscoliosis progresses, there will be a decrease in the height of a patient, which is one parameter than can be used to follow the course of the disease. Pain is the primary complaint. Generally, there is no neural compression.

DIFFERENTIAL DIAGNOSIS

The majority of patients do not develop a significant kyphoscoliosis but present with pain secondary to a vertebral body compression fracture.

TABLE 8–2. Causes of Osteopenia

Genetic	Osteogenesis imperfecta
	Homocystinuria
Endocrine	Hypogonadism
	Hyperadrenocorticism
	Hyperthyroidism
	Hyperparathyroidism
	Acromegaly
Nutritional	Calcium deficiency
	Protein deficiency
	Ascorbic acid deficiency
	Intestinal malabsorption
Drug-Induced	Heparin
	Anticonvulsants
	Methotrexate
	Ethanol
Miscellaneous	Metabolic acidosis
	Rheumatoid arthritis
	Trauma
	Disease

There are many entities that can have a similar presentation, but three are quite common and should be specifically ruled out in each instance. Tumor, especially a solitary myeloma, is relatively common in the older age group. Osteomalacia is also prevalent in the older population as a result of their dietary habits. Finally, an endocrine abnormality is quite possible. This would include hyperparathyroidism, hyperthyroidism, and Cushing's disease.

It should be appreciated that osteomalacia, endocrine abnormalities, and tumors, as well as osteoporosis, can all be included under the general heading of osteopenia, which is defined as abnormal bone loss.[13] When the physician is faced with a patient who has increased bone loss, the patient should be considered osteopenic. Only when the other possibilities are excluded should he be labeled osteoporotic. Osteoporosis is a diagnosis of exclusion. Table 8–2 is a complete list of the identifiable causes of osteopenia.[24]

RADIOGRAPHIC AND LABORATORY FINDINGS

Osteoporosis has no definitive radiographic or laboratory findings. The studies that are routinely obtained are to rule out the other common causes of osteopenia.

Radiographically, the lateral projection of the spine will yield the most information. Other views, including the AP and obliques, are helpful in excluding entities such as arthritis and neoplasm.

Osteoporosis results in a decrease in bone density in the vertebral body. Approximately 30 per cent of the bone mineral must be lost before a standard lateral x-ray will show an increase in radiolucency.[12] Also, all of the other osteopenic conditions will decrease bone density. Thus, increased radiolucency, although consistent with osteoporosis, is not specific.

If the mineral loss is severe, the strength of the vertebral body is decreased and a change in shape will result. Wedging and compression of the vertebral body are the most common deformities.[8] Wedging is a reduction in the height of the anterior border of the vertebral body as compared with the posterior border, which remains normal. Compression is a reduction in height of the entire vertebral body including the posterior border. The etiology of both wedging and compression is a fracture. The different changes that can occur in the x-ray of a vertebral body may help in arriving at a diagnosis.

In osteoporosis, wedging and compression are most frequently seen (Figs. 8–1, 8–2). Biconcavity of the vertebral bodies may be found in osteoporosis, but the borders are irregular and it is not common. This reveals that osteoporotic bone is brittle and fractures easily. The changes in osteoporotic vertebrae are usually unevenly distributed along the spine.[6] Characteristically, no two affected vertebrae are alike, and sometimes affected vertebrae may be separated by one that is normal.

There are no specific laboratory findings diagnostic of osteoporosis.

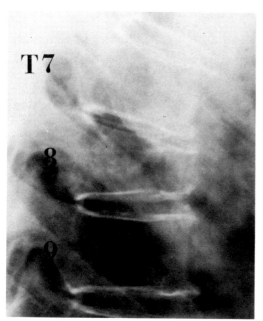

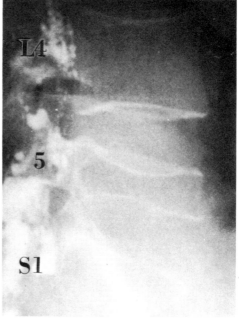

Figure 8–1. Wedging of T8, which demonstrates an intact posterior border of the vertebral body with collapse of the anterior boarder. (From Rothman, R. H., and Simeone, F. A.: The Spine, 1st ed. Philadelphia, W. B. Saunders Co., 1975.)

Figure 8–2. Compression of L5 with collapse of both the anterior and posterior borders of the vertebral body. (From Rothman, R. H., and Simeone, F. A.: The Spine, 1st ed. Philadelphia, W. B. Saunders Co., 1975.)

The tests that are done are to rule out the other major causes of osteopenia. These include osteomalacia, tumors (multiple myeloma), hyperparathyroidism, hyperthyroidism, and Cushing's disease.

TREATMENT

The goal in the treatment of osteoporosis is to prevent the abnormal loss of mineral. To date, this has been unsuccessful, since the actual etiology of osteoporosis is unknown.

The treatment of osteoporosis of the spine is basically symptomatic. Disabling pain is usually present only during an acute fracture episode. Bed rest and appropriate analgesics are indicated. Elderly patients do need aid in their daily care, and many times it is necessary to hospitalize these people for the initial treatment period. Fortunately, the fractures seem to heal without difficulty.

A custom-fitted elastic corset will give good support to these patients during the acutely painful fracture episodes. They are also helpful on a long-term basis. Rigid metal braces are not well received and may cause problems.

Between fractures, patients should be encouraged to exercise, and it is surprising how well these people can perform with only a little encouragement. Stationary bicycle riding and swimming are the safest and most satisfactory exercises. Patients with severe osteoporosis seem to be prone to accidental falls. A cane is quite helpful, and soft rubber–heeled shoes appear to decrease spinal impact and increase floor traction. Unfortunately, fractures seem to appear at unpredictable intervals, and the patient should realize that this is a life-long problem.

There is no successful medical treatment for these patients. The therapies that are used are based on the supposition that osteoporosis is a disorder of calcium homeostasis.[25] It is felt that if a positive calcium balance is produced, the progress of osteoporosis may be decreased and, it is hoped, even prevented. Unfortunately, this has not been the case to date.

Several treatment regimens are currently used. The older modalities are high calcium and phosphorus intake, sex hormones, and vitamin D. The new therapies include calcitonin, diphosphonates, and fluoride ion. It is uncertain which of these is the most beneficial. Our preference is to treat these patients on a long-term basis with 1.5 gm. of calcium a day, plus 50,000 units of vitamin D twice a week. Estrogens are used on a short-term basis (90 days) to control pain.

OSTEOMALACIA

Osteomalacia is a disturbance in the formation of bone in the adult skeleton caused by the failure of the deposition of bone salts within the organic matrix. The ratio of the mineral to the osteoid is decreased.[26]

Pathophysiology

In osteomalacia, there is a failure of calcification of the matrix. The primary etiology behind this unmineralized osteoid is varied, but the basic deficit is that there is not enough mineral (calcium or phosphorus) available for crystal formation.

Table 8–3 outlines the major causes.[5] Abnormal vitamin D metabolism or deficiency states are the most common problems in the elderly.

The usual sequence of events in the older patients is that there is a decrease in calcium absorption from the gastrointestinal tract caused by either a deficient diet or abnormal gastrointestinal function. A transient fall of serum calcium results, which leads to a stimulation of parathyroid hormone and a subsequent increase in bone resorption. In response to the bone loss, osteoblasts will manufacture osteoid, but if the calcium deprivation is long-term, there will not be enough crystals to mineralize the normal osteoid. The ratio of the mineral to osteoid is decreased, and the bone becomes soft.

Signs and Symptoms

The clinical features of osteomalacia are varied. The patient may initially complain of muscular weakness, inability to walk stairs, and vague localized pains. Sometimes muscle cramps are a prominent feature, and this is probably secondary to hypocalcemia. As the disease progresses, kyphoscoliosis may become very prominent and will generally be associated

---

TABLE 8–3. Causes of Osteomalacia

Deficiency States
  Vitamin D
  Calcium
  Phosphorus
  Chelators

GI Absorption Defects
  Gastric abnormalities
  Biliary disease
  Enteric absorptive defects

Renal Tubular Defects
  Proximal tubular lesions
  Distal tubular lesions
  Proximal and distal tubular lesions

Renal Osteodystrophy

Osteomalacia Associated with other Conditions
  Fibrous dysplasia
  Neurofibromatosis
  Soft tissue and bone neoplasms such as giant cell tumor or nonossifying fibroma
  Anticonvulsant medication

---

with pain. There are no specific signs and symptoms that are diagnostic of osteomalacia.

RADIOGRAPHIC AND LABORATORY FINDINGS

In the spine, the most common radiographic finding is biconcavity of the vertebral bodies (Fig. 8–3). This has been referred to as "codfish vertebra."[19] The curves are smooth because the bone is softer than normal but not brittle. Vertebrae along the course of the spine are usually affected to the same extent. The lumbar vertebrae may be involved more severely than the thoracic vertebrae, but there is a smooth progression throughout the spine.

The other significant radiographic finding in osteomalacia is pseudofractures. A pseudofracture is a transverse radiolucency that arises spontaneously.[23] They do not heal until the underlying defect is corrected. Pseudofractures occur in approximately one third of all patients with osteomalacia and are usually found in the ribs and pelvic rami. The defects are often bilateral. These pseudofractures are often referred to as Looser's lines or Milkman's fractures.

Laboratory data will reveal a low-normal serum calcium level, a slightly depressed serum inorganic phosphate level, and a mildly elevated alkaline phosphatase level. These values, especially the serum calcium, are not strikingly abnormal because of the role of parathyroid hormone. This

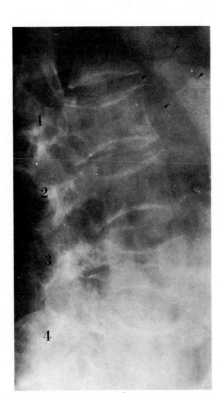

Figure 8–3. Osteomalacia of lumbar spine demonstrating biconcavity and two pseudofractures in a rib (arrows). (From Rothman, R. H., and Simeone, F. A.: The Spine, 1st ed. Philadelphia, W. B. Saunders Co., 1975.)

hormone will keep the serum level of calcium relatively close to normal at the expense of bone calcium.

A 24-hour urine study will demonstrate a calcium content of less than 75 mg. per day in 95 per cent of patients with osteomalacia. This is relatively specific for osteomalacia and thus is an effective screening test that can be used on an outpatient basis.[27]

The only way to definitively diagnose osteomalacia is to perform a bone biopsy.[20] The specimen, usually obtained from the iliac crest, should not be decalcified; this must be stressed. A positive biopsy specimen will show an increase in the width of the osteoid seams. The normal osteoid border is 15 μ wide, whereas in patients with osteomalacia, the border is over 20 μ wide and lacks a mineralization front.

DIFFERENTIAL DIAGNOSIS

Osteomalacia is one of the osteopenic conditions, and the various possibilities that have to be considered are outlined in Table 8–2. As the physician evaluates osteopenia, each of these entities must be ruled out. It should be appreciated that once the general diagnosis of osteomalacia is made, the next step is to pinpoint its etiology. This is usually either a deficiency problem, gastrointestinal absorption defect, or a renal problem. However, there are several conditions that can be associated with or cause osteomalacia that need to be remembered. Most of these conditions, such as that caused by anticoagulation medication, interfere with vitamin D metabolism.[22]

TREATMENT

The correct management of osteomalacia depends on the underlying disorder. For example, if steatorrhea is preventing the absorption of vitamin D, the gastrointestinal disorder needs primary treatment. In general, the problem of soft bone can be handled with 1.5 gm. of calcium per day plus 50,000 units of vitamin D twice a week. The serum calcium level should be determined on a regular basis to prevent hypercalcemia. Unlike osteoporosis, in which fracture healing is normal, the pseudofractures in osteomalacia will not heal until the primary conditions are eliminated. Symptomatic support of the back with a brace is helpful while the impaired bone healing defect is corrected.

HYPERPARATHYROIDISM

Primary hyperparathyroidism is an increase in the secretion of parathyroid hormone. In 80 per cent of the cases, a single parathyroid adenoma is responsible. Clear cell hyperplasia occurs 15 per cent of the time, and cancer is the etiologic factor in the remaining 5 per cent.[29]

Secondary hyperparathyroidism is the increased secretion of parathyroid hormone as a response to another pathophysiologic problem. These other disorders result in calcium deficiency states and are generally associated with abnormal vitamin D metabolism.

PATHOPHYSIOLOGY

Parathyroid hormone affects the bones, kidneys, and intestines to raise the serum calcium level. As calcium is reabsorbed from the bone, osteitis fibrosa cystica may result. Osteitis fibrosa cystica is the replacement of normal bone with fibrous tissue and surrounding osseous metaplasia.[11] Brown tumors may be found in far advanced hyperparathyroidism. Brown tumors are bone cysts that are filled with vascular fibrous tissue interspersed with hemosiderin macrophages and giant cells.

Today, most patients with primary hyperparathyroidism never develop osteitis fibrosa cystica because the disease is usually diagnosed early in its course. The patients seek medical attention because of kidney stones or the systemic effects of hypercalcemia. Patients with hyperthyroidism secondary to chronic renal failure do seem to be more prone to developing osteitis fibrosa cystica. This is a result of the chronicity of the renal disease and the inability to cure the basic disease process.

SIGNS AND SYMPTOMS

Hyperparathyroidism is twice as common in females who are between the third and fifth decade of life. The onset is generally insidious with lethargy, loss of appetite, nausea, vomiting, and polydipsia as the main complaints. Pancreatitis and recurrent renal stones are associated problems.

The spine is variably affected in hyperparathyroidism. The general disease may be quite severe with only mild back involvement, or the back may be the patient's most troublesome area. The chief complaint is pain with a developing kyphosis. With severe vertebral body collapse, there may be significant loss of height. The kyphosis is usually evenly distributed throughout the spine and can include the cervical region. Finally, the vertebral collapse may be quite progressive, but significant pain is not always an accompanying factor.

RADIOGRAPHIC AND LABORATORY FINDINGS

Radiographically, the lateral view of the spine is the most informative. The vertebrae are compressed and slightly wedged. With long-standing disease, end-plate sclerosis will occur, producing a picture of what is commonly referred to as a "rugger jersey" spine[31] (Figs. 8–4, 8–5). As the spine involvement progresses, severe wedging with significant angulation may occur. Other radiographic changes include subperiosteal resorption,

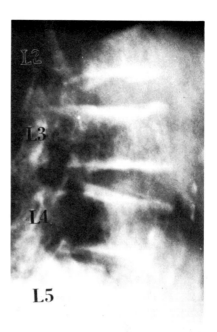

Figure 8–4. Lumbar spine of patient with long-standing primary hyperparathyroidism. End-plate sclerosis is present leading to the "rugger jersey" description. (From Rothman, R. H., and Simeone, F. A.: The Spine, 1st ed. Philadelphia, W. B. Saunders Co., 1975.)

especially in the phalanges, a mottled appearance of the skull, and cysts in the long bones.

In the laboratory studies, the most consistent abnormality is an elevated alkaline phosphatase level. The serum calcium level is elevated,

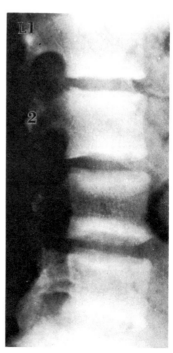

Figure 8–5. Patient with secondary hyperparathyroidism due to renal disease. X-ray demonstrates typical "rugger jersey" appearance. (From Rothman, R. H., and Simeone, F. A.: The Spine, 1st ed. Philadelphia, W. B. Saunders Co., 1975.)

and the serum phosphorus level is low. The percentage of trabecular reabsorption of phosphate (TRP) is 70 per cent or less.[15] It should be noted that many diseases increase serum calcium, but only primary hyperparathyroidism causes a decreased TRP. Recently, direct assay of the concentration of parathyroid hormone has come into use, and the hormone will be elevated in both primary and secondary hyperparathyroidism. Finally, if a bone biopsy is performed, the specimen will reveal increased fibrous tissue with osteoblasts and osteoclasts surrounding the same trabeculae.

DIFFERENTIAL DIAGNOSIS

The diagnosis of hyperparathyroidism can usually be made by hand x-rays demonstrating subperiosteal erosion in the phalanges and a high alkaline phosphatase level. The difficulty comes in distinguishing between primary and secondary hyperparathyroidism. The physician must obtain the necessary studies to rule in or rule out the various entities listed in Table 8–3.

On x-ray, a rugger jersey spine can be seen, caused by primary hyperparathyroidism, renal osteodystrophy (secondary hyperparathyroidism), and osteopetrosis. The possible diagnoses in a patient with wedge compression fractures, hypercalcemia, and an increased alkaline phosphatase level include primary hyperparathyroidism, malignancy (either primary or secondary), or immobilization. Each of these problems must be considered and ruled out with an organized work-up.

TREATMENT

Surgical intervention is the principal treatment of primary hyperparathyroidism. Once the source of the increased parathyroid hormone is removed, the skeleton lesions will usually heal. There may be some residual limb deformity and, if symptomatic, it can be appropriately corrected.

Secondary hyperparathyroidism is best approached by treating the underlying cause. In some cases, such as chronic renal failure, the urinary etiology cannot be cured, and the resultant problems have to be handled symptomatically. Regarding the spine, this means external support and analgesic medication as necessary.

PAGET'S DISEASE

Paget's disease is a focal bone disorder characterized initially by excessive resorption and, subsequently, formation of abnormal bone. This abnormal bone consists of a mosaic pattern of lamellar bone that is associated with extensive focal vascularity and increased fibrous tissue in the adjacent marrow.[7]

PATHOPHYSIOLOGY

The etiology of Paget's disease is unknown. It is believed that Paget's disease evolves through three phases. The first phase is a focal intensive resorption of existing bone. This is an osteolytic or destructive process. On a biopsy specimen, one will see scalloped resorptive spaces filled with osteoclasts that may contain as many as one hundred nuclei. The second phase is an increase in both bone formation and resorption. This is termed the "mixed state." The last phase is sclerotic or osteoblastic. The osteon unit organization is lost, and there is a failure of the remodeling process. A thick woven bone is produced in a mosaic pattern. Although these three phases are described in sequence, they may all occur at once.[14]

Metabolically, there is an overall increase in bone turnover with normal serum levels of calcium, phosphorus, and parathyroid hormone. There is an increase in the urinary excretion of hydroxyproline, which reflects the increase in collagen breakdown. There is also a high alkaline phosphatase level secondary to the increased osteoblastic activity.

SIGNS AND SYMPTOMS

Any bone may be affected by Paget's disease. The most common sites are the spine, pelvis, skull, femora, and tibias. Pain in the involved bone is the predominant complaint, although many patients are asymptomatic.

Most patients have some degree of spine involvement. Along with pain, dorsal kyphosis can be a major problem.[3] Vertebral body fractures do occur, but they usually heal without difficulty. Sarcomatous degeneration does occur in the spine but accounts for only about 3 per cent of Paget's disease sarcomas. A sudden increase in pain is the major complaint when sarcomas arise.

Neurologic compression can occur. It is most common in the thoracic spine where the canal diameter is the smallest, although it can occur at any level.[18] The clinical effects depend on the level of the disease. Usually, weakness and numbness develop gradually in both legs with no sharp sensory level, since compression is spread out over several vertebrae. Spinal cord decompression is quite successful in these patients. Infrequently, cord compression appears suddenly. This is usually a result of a single vertebral body collapse and is an indication for surgical intervention. Finally, nerve root compression from foraminal encroachment can occur in the lumbar spine. It should be appreciated that these neurologic problems associated with Paget's disease are rare.

RADIOGRAPHIC AND LABORATORY FINDINGS

As with the other metabolic diseases, the lateral x-rays of the spine are the most informative. The vertebral body is usually expanded, and its appearance varies with the stage of the disease. Usually, the vertebral cortex is thickened, especially along the perimeter of the body. The

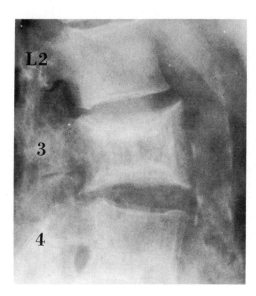

Figure 8–6. L3 vertebra demonstrating picture-frame appearance in a patient with Paget's disease. (From Rothman, R. H., and Simeone, F. A.: The Spine, 1st ed. Philadelphia, W. B. Saunders Co., 1975.)

resultant appearance may be similar to a picture frame that is filled with coarse, irregular bone[30] (Fig. 8–6). Depending on the balance between formation and resorption, different degrees of sclerosis may be visualized. The most extreme sclerosis is commonly referred to as an ivory vertebra and is usually an isolated finding.

The most common laboratory abnormality is an elevated serum alkaline phosphatase level. This is a rough reflection of the increased osteoblastic activity. The urinary hydroxyproline level is also elevated. Both of these values correlate fairly well with the activity of the disease and can be helpful in following a patient's response to treatment. The serum calcium, phosphorus, and parathyroid hormone levels are normal. Occasionally, the acid phosphatase level may be elevated, which can pose a problem in distinguishing Paget's disease from metastatic prostate carcinoma.

TREATMENT

The medical treatment of Paget's disease is still evolving. At present, suppression of disease activity and symptomatic relief are possible, but actual improvement in the bone structure has not been achieved.[32] A number of therapeutic agents are available and include calcitonin, EHDP (diphosphonate disodiumethymate), and Metromycin. At present, calcitonin appears to be the safest and most suitable agent for general use.

Bone pain of the spine is best treated initially by anti-inflammatory medications. If the discomfort is not relieved, treatment with one of the previously mentioned agents should be tried. Fractures and kyphosis are best treated symptomatically with rest and support. Finally, neurologic compromise, whether it be of the cord, cauda equina, or nerve root, should be surgically decompressed. If for any reason this is not possible, medical treatment should be instituted. Again, calcitonin seems to be the drug of choice and on occasion will lead to surprising improvement.

GOUT

Gout principally affects the appendicular joints; however, it does on occasion involve the axial skeleton. The main focus of urate deposition is the sacroiliac joints,[21] although the intervertebral disc spaces can also be affected.

Historically, all of these patients will suffer from peripheral gouty arthritis for a number of years, with the average age being greater than 50.[20] The majority of these individuals will be under active treatment. The primary complaint is the gradual onset of nonradiating low back pain. The symptoms of these patients are secondary to chronic gouty arthritis. In contrast, a few patients will have sudden onset of pain and will be found to have acute gouty arthritis of the sacroiliac joint.

The physical examination is nonspecific. Those patients with an acute attack will have a stiff spine, little if any motion, and significant spasm. Any movement of the spine will produce severe discomfort. The physician may be able to reproduce the pain on the involved side by flexing, abducting, and externally rotating the hip.

When the sacroiliac articulation is initially involved, an x-ray will demonstrate narrowing or obliteration of the joint space with sclerosis of the joint margins (Fig. 8–7). Discrete subchondral cysts can be found on both sides of the joint. As the disease progresses, gross irregularity of the joint surface can occur with marginal osteophytes.

To reach the proper diagnosis, a physician must have a high index of

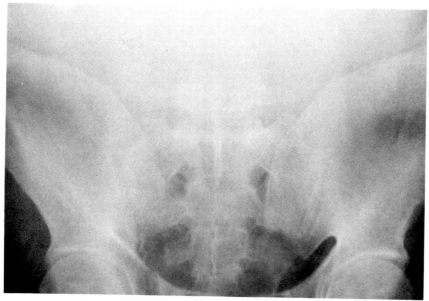

Figure 8–7. Gouty involvement of right S1 joint. The joint margins are indistinct with sclerosis.

suspicion. Whenever an older patient presents with acute low back pain, tophaceous involvement of the sacroiliac joint should be considered. As already mentioned, these patients will have had gout for a number of years, and having most likely been under treatment for a significant period of time, a blood uric acid level will not necessarily be abnormal. Synovial fluid for analysis is difficult to obtain from the sacroliac joint. There are no easily available tests, x-rays, or signs that are pathognomonic for gout.

Practially speaking, the best approach for an older patient with a positive history of gout and back pain is a trial dose of colchicine. If in fact the patient does have gout, a dramatic response will follow this therapy. After the acute symptoms are under control, the patient's medication can be appropriately regulated.

REFERENCES

1. Adams, P., Davies, G. T., and Sweetnam, P.: Osteoporosis and the effects of aging on bone mass in elderly men and women. Q. J. Med., *39*:601, 1970.
2. Aegertir, E., and Kirkpatrick, J. A.: Orthopaedic diseases. Philadelphia, W. B. Saunders Co., 1975.
3. Aldren-Turner, J. W.: The spinal complication of Paget's disease. Brain, *63*:321, 1940.
4. Arnold, J. S., Bartley, M. H., Tont, S. A., and Jenkins, D. P.: Skeletal changes in aging and disease. Clin. Orthop., *49*:17, 1966.
5. Avioli, L., and Haddad, J. G.: Vitamin D: Current concepts. Metabolism, *22*:507, 1973.
6. Barnett, E., and Nordin, B. E. C.: The radiologic diagnosis of osteoporosis. A new approach. Clin. Radiol., *11*:166, 1962.
7. Barry, H. C.: Paget's Disease of Bone. London, Livingstone, 1969.
8. Bick, E. M., and Copel, J. W.: Fractures of vertebrae in the aged. Geriatrics, *5*:74, 1950.
9. Caldwell, R. A.: Observation in the indicence, etiology and pathology of senile osteoporosis. J. Clin. Pathol., *15*:421, 1962.
10. Chalmers, J., Conacher, V. D. H., Gardner, D. L., et al.: Osteomalacia: a common disease in elderly women. J. Bone Joint Surg., *49B*:403, 1967.
11. Dent, C. E.: Some problems of hyperparathyroidism. Brit. Med. J., *2*:1419, 1495, 1962.
12. Dent, C. E., and Hodson, C. H.: Radiological changes associated with certain metabolic bone diseases. Symposium. Generalized softening of bone due to metabolic causes. Brit. J. Radiol., *27*:605, 1954.
13. Dent, C. E., and Watson, L.: Osteoporosis. Postgrad. Med. J., *42* (Suppl.):582, 1966.
14. Dickson, D. D., Camp, J. D., and Ghormley, R. K.: Osteitis deformans: Paget's disease of the bone. Radiology, *44*:449, 1945.
15. Fourman, P., and Royer, P.: Calcium metabolism and the bone. Oxford, Blackwell Scientific Publications, 1968.
16. Frame, B.: Metabolic bone disease as a cause of neck ache and back ache. Proceedings of conference in neckache and backache in association with neurologic surgery. Springfield, Charles C Thomas Pub., 1970.
17. Harris, W. H., and Heaney, R. P.: Skeletal renewal and metabolic bone disease. N. Engl. J. Med., *28*:193, 253, 303, 1969.
18. Hartman, J. T., and John, D. F.: Paget's disease of the spine with cord and nerve root compression. J. Bone Joint Surg., *48A*:1079, 1966.
19. Hurxthal, I. M.: Measurement of anterior vertebral compressions and biconcave vertebrae. Am. J. Roentgenol., *53*:635, 1968.
20. Lipson, R. I., and Slocumb, C. H.: The progressive nature of gout with inadequate therapy. Arthritis Rheum., *8*:80, February 1965.
21. Malawista, S. E., Aeegmiller, J. E., Hathaway, B. E., and Skoloff, L.: Sacroiliac gout. JAMA, *194*:9, 1965.
22. Mankin, H. J.: Rickets, osteomalacia and renal osteodystrophy. J. Bone Joint Surg., *56A*:101, 352, 1974.
23. Milkman, L. A.: Pseudofractures (hunger osteopathy, late rickets, osteomalacia). Am. J. Roentgenol., *24*:29, 1930.

24. Morgan, D. B.: Osteomalacia, renal osteodystrophy and osteoporosis. Springfield, Charles C Thomas Pub., 1973.
25. Nordin, B. E. C.: Clinical significance and pathogenesis of osteoporosis. Br. Med. J., *1*:571, 1971.
26. Nordin, B. E. C.: Osteomalacia, osteoporosis and calcium deficiency. Clin. Orthop., *17*:235, 1960.
27. Nordin, B. E. C.: Hodgkinson, A., and Peacock, M.: The measurement and the meaning of urinary calcium. Clin. Orthop., *52*:293, 1967.
28. Nordin, B. E. C., and Smith, D. A.: Diagnostic procedures in disorders of calcium metabolism. London, J. A. Churchill, Ltd., 1965.
29. Pyrah, L. N., Hodgkinson, A., and Anderson, C. K.: Primary hyperparathyroidism. Br. J. Surg., *53*:234, 1966.
30. Schreiber, M. H., and Richardson, L. A.: Paget's disease confined to one lumbar vertebra. Am. J. Roentgenol., *90*:1271, 1963.
31. Steinbach, H. L.: Roentgenology of the skeleton in the aged. Radiol. Clin. North Am., *3*:277, 1965.
32. Trotter, M., Broman, G. E., and Peterson, R. R.: Densities of bone of white and Negro skeletons. J. Bone Joint Surg., *42A*:50, 1960.
33. Urist, M. P., Gurvey, M. S., and Fareed, D. O.: Long term observations on aged women with pathologic osteoporosis. Clin. Orthop., *70*:3, 1970.
34. Wu, K., and Frost, H. M.: Bone formation in osteoporosis. Arch. Pathol., *88*:508, 1969.

Chapter 9

SURGICAL TECHNIQUES

INTRODUCTION

Of all the surgical endeavors within the realm of orthopedic surgery, none can produce the predictable and satisfying level of excellence that is seen with modern spinal surgery. The indications are now clearly understood, the selection of operation is simple, and the surgical techniques are easily mastered. If the surgeon stays within the accepted guidelines and is judicious in the selection of patients, surgery of the spine can be most gratifying for both the treating physician and the patient.

INDICATIONS FOR SURGERY

If the various nonsurgical treatment modalities discussed in the chapter on conservative management are not successful, surgery becomes the "conservative management" of choice.

Profound or Progressive Neurologic Deficit

The most dramatic presentation of an acute disc herniation is the cauda equina syndrome, which is the most certain indication for immediate surgical intervention. If bowel, bladder, and sexual function are to be preserved, immediate decompression of the cauda equina is imperative. The complex interplay of compression, edema, and vascular insult to the cauda equina secondary to disc herniation alone or in combination with surgical intervention makes a prediction as to outcome difficult. The temporal framework within which the syndrome develops and within which surgical treatment is realized are also factors that affect the prognosis. In any event, the rarity of spontaneous recovery of sexual and sphincter function[5] makes myelographic definition and rapid surgical decompression of paramount importance.

Motor weakness requires more judgment in terms of urgency as a criterion for surgical intervention. Because of their functional importance, acute complete paralysis of the quadriceps muscle or of the dorsiflexors of the foot is an indication for surgical decompression of the involved spinal nerves. The more prolonged the pressure on the spinal nerve and the more intense the compression, the less likely is the return of function. It should be stated, however, that this guideline is not absolute, and in the author's experience, several cases with these circumstances have been seen in which the recommended decompression was not undertaken and the patient had complete restoration of function with the passage of time.

In Weber's[8] excellent prospective study, the degree of residual paresis was similar in the surgically treated and conservatively treated groups after three years. It is possible that the surgical results were compromised by an initial period of nonoperative management. The authors agree with Weber that with acute profound motor weakness, decompression should be performed as soon as possible. When lesser degrees of motor weakness are present and the situation is subacute, judgment must be exercised as to when surgery should be recommended. If the weakness is mild to moderate and compatible with adequate function of the extremity, a period of observation and conservative treatment is indicated. This is particularly true in subacute and chronic situations. However, if the motor weakness is progressive in nature and becomes significant in terms of function, surgical intervention is mandatory.

Sensory and reflex changes are helpful in terms of diagnosis but are not in themselves indications for surgical intervention and are of no prognostic value in predicting the ultimate outcome of the disease. Weber found sensory dysfunction in nearly 46 per cent of his total series of patients after four years. The abnormalities that were encountered existed either prior to treatment or developed subsequent to either surgical or conservative management. It is interesting to note that no patient was disabled because of sensory deficits. Similarly, a diminution or loss of reflex in the face of lessening pain would certainly not be an indication for surgery.

Unrelenting Sciatica

Occasionally, an acute attack of sciatica will fail to respond to all forms of conservative treatment. The exact time after which surgery should be recommended will vary from patient to patient according to their pain tolerance, emotional stability, and the demands of their socioeconomic environment. In general, the authors do not recommend surgical consideration in acute sciatica before a period of four to six weeks has elapsed. Since 80 per cent of Weber's nonsurgically managed group showed "good" or "fair" results within three months, observation is justified for this period of time. If the period of conservative treatment results in little or no improvement, surgical intervention should be undertaken. Further procrastination will adversely affect the results of surgery.

Recurrent Episodes of Sciatica

After an initial successful course of conservative treatment, certain individuals will have recurrent sciatica that becomes incapacitating. There may be a complete absence of symptoms between the acute episodes, or low-grade sciatica may continue to a greater or lesser extent. If the recurrent episodes are not disabling and if the intensity of the symptoms is within the patient's emotional tolerance, persistent conservative therapy is indicated. However, if the frequency and intensity of the attacks are severe enough to interfere with the individual's ability to be gainfully employed and enjoy normal activities of daily living, surgery should be undertaken. In general, the authors would consider surgery only after three recurrent sciatic episodes, but there is variation in this regard.

Personality Factors

Care must be taken to evaluate both the emotional stability of these patients and their reaction to pain. A person who continues to have minor symptoms with conservative therapy but who has an overwhelming emotional reaction to the pain will usually do poorly even after surgery, particularly if an element of hostility is present.

However, the authors emphasize that this admonition is not proposed in order to differentiate the "functional" from the "organic" back pain patient. Indeed, it would be naive to overlook the reciprocal interaction between the patient's somatic and emotional states. Rather, effective management of this disabling episode of pain may rest on coincident psychotherapeutic support, carefully monitored antidepressant medication, or both.[4]

An efficient and rapid psychiatric assessment[10] can be elicited using the following points of subjectivity:

1. Has the patient's pain precipitated adverse mood changes? (That is, are the patient's "spirits down?")

2. Has there been an onset of vegetative behavioral changes (appetite alterations, sleep disturbances, and diminution in libido)?

3. Has the pain created problems at home or work?

4. Has the patient demonstrated an appropriate response to management thus far?

The use of the MMPI Conversion 5 profile as demonstrated by Hanvick,[2] its modified form,[9] or the pain drawing screening test introduced by Ransford and others[7] may shed some light on the psychiatric factors that are involved. However, in and of themselves, these ancillary studies are more a temporal indication of the patient's intensity of the fear of pain than a statement as to the etiology of that pain.[1, 6]

If there is any uncertainty as to the emotional stability of the patient, psychiatric consultation is mandatory. This is not to say that all patients with emotional problems, particularly those with long-standing pain, should be denied surgical relief. It has been well demonstrated that long-standing pain will lead to depression even in basically stable individuals and that depression will sometimes lift after the pain is alleviated. In general, it is a good rule of thumb to treat the emotional factors prior to making a surgical decision. More often than not, intolerable pain becomes quite tolerable once depression has lifted.

In most instances, surgery will be undertaken for the relief of sciatic pain, and its effectiveness will depend on the discovery and relief of pressure upon the neural elements. Ideally, every operative procedure performed to relieve sciatica would reveal mechanical compromise of the nerve roots. This is occasionally not the case, and in these instances, surgery will often fail. One might assume that failure to discover mechanical compression is a result of one of two factors, either an inadequate exploration or a nonmechanical cause of the sciatica. The first-mentioned factor may be remedied by a more thorough exploration and a more complete understanding of the pathology. The nonmechanical sciatica can best be appreciated by an analysis of those factors present in the preoperative evaluation that best correlate with the presence or absence of demonstrable nerve root compression. The most thorough study in this regard is that of Hirsh[3] in a review of approximately 3000 low back operations. He found that the most significant preoperative factors in the determination of mechanical paraspinal nerve compression were (1) a well-defined neurologic deficit, (2) a positive myelogram, and (3) a positive straight leg raising test.

When all of these factors are present, surgery will usually uncover mechanical compression and will be followed by a good result. If one or more of these factors are absent, much deliberation should take place before surgery is undertaken. This is not to say that one should not recommend surgery in the absence of a positive myelogram or neurologic deficit but that careful evaluation of these cases should be made. If, for instance, the patient has a well-defined neurologic deficit (such as an absent Achilles reflex), a positive straight leg raising test, and a positive contralateral straight leg raising test, the surgeon might expect to find a herniated L5 disc compromising the S1 spinal nerve, despite a normal Pantopaque myelogram. However, if two out of three critical factors are missing, such as a positive myelogram and neurologic deficit, one might well expect a negative exploration and failure to relieve the sciatica postoperatively.

The authors have recently modified these guidelines as follows. In order to predict mechanical root compression, the patient must have (1) *either* a positive tension sign *or* a neurologic deficit *and* (2) a correlative finding on contrast studies (metrizamide myelography or epidural venography). With the use of both water-soluble myelography and epidural venography, both of which are highly sensitive, it would be most unusual for us to undertake surgical exploration without radiographic confirmation of root compression. False-negative studies are becoming increasingly rare.

SELECTION OF THE OPERATION

Acute Disc Herniation

In most individuals with acute disc herniations, the primary compelling symptom that leads to surgery is sciatica. Although the patient may have had many years of preceding troublesome but tolerable back pain, the leg symptoms ultimately will force him toward surgery. In individuals such as this, limited laminectomy with excision of the herniated material as well as excision of the nucleus of the abnormal disc is the procedure of choice. The approach may be limited, and in cases with a wide interlaminar space, little or no bone need be removed. It is essential that the nerve root be completely explored well out through the foramen and be free of all external pressure and tension at the termination of the procedure.

Chronic Disc Degeneration and Spinal Stenosis

BACK PAIN ONLY

Most individuals with chronic disc degeneration and back pain can be managed effectively with nonoperative treatment. The authors advocate a very conservative posture in regard to surgical treatment of patients with disc degeneration and back pain only. The rationale for this is that disc degeneration often becomes a diffuse process throughout the entire lumbar spine with the passage of time, and furthermore, it is extremely difficult to ascertain which of the several levels may be the source of the patient's pain. Occasionally, an individual will develop severe incapacitating back pain that is intractable to medical therapy and is clearly limited to one or two disc spaces. These individuals will obtain relief through arthrodesis of the spine. The procedure of choice is a bilateral spine fusion from the affected level to the sacrum. When surgery is undertaken for this type of diagnostic category, a fusion of L4 to the sacrum is usually performed. A bone graft should not be placed in the midline over the lamina, as it will lead to thickening of the lamina with the possible late formation of spinal stenosis (see Fig. 9–7). The diagnostic entity of spinal stenosis after midline spinal fusion is seen with greater frequency as experience with spinal fusion increases.

BACK AND LEG PAIN

Patients with chronic disc degeneration will present with a wide variety of ratios of back to leg pain. One extreme is the individual with florid sciatica and negligible back pain. This individual requires decompression only if it can be accomplished without the creation of instability during the operation. If a strong component of back pain is present, stabilization should be undertaken at the same time, with a bilateral lateral spinal fusion incorporating the degenerated levels down through the sacrum. The combined procedure of decompression and fusion is also indicated if iatrogenic instability is created (bilateral foraminotomy at one level) or if demonstrable radiographic instability is evident. It should be noted that a combined laminectomy and fusion is rarely performed, since patients with predominant back pain are generally poor candidates for surgery; furthermore, it is rarely necessary to render a spine unstable surgically when performing a decompression.

The type of pathologic condition will dictate the extent and type of decompression required. If midline ridging is the only abnormality present and the nerve roots are free in the foramen, complete laminectomy of the affected levels with preservation of the facet joints will suffice. If there is an extrusion of disc material, it obviously should be removed, but this is not usually the case in end-stage disc degeneration. The disc space need not be entered in the majority of these individuals, since little nuclear material will be present.

Although the symptoms may be unilateral, the authors would advise performing a complete bilateral laminectomy to prevent contralateral symptomatology in the future. If there is foraminal encroachment, a complete foraminotomy is indicated. If a narrow lateral recess is present, it must be unroofed completely out to the pedicle. When possible, the lateral portion of the facet joint is maintained intact. Often this is not possible, particularly on the patient's symptomatic side; if so, complete removal of the facets and complete foraminotomy should be undertaken.

In certain individuals, even after foraminotomy and unroofing of the lateral recesses, the nerve root will still be tightly tethered around a pedicle that has undergone a relative descent during disc degeneration. In these individuals, excision of the pedicle is necessary. Occasionally, a lateral herniation or the presence of an aberrant ligament, such as the corporo-transverse ligament, will cause nerve root compression distal to the foramen. These sources of nerve root compression must be corrected.

In the majority of patients with chronic disc degeneration, there should be a minimum of two levels of decompression, that is, at L5 and L4; in developmental spinal stenosis, a minimum of three levels are decompressed, extending up to L3. The decision as to how far craniad to proceed with decompression will also depend upon the operative findings, and we would not hesitate to advocate complete lumbar decompression from L1 to L5 if the pathologic condition warrants it.

It should be reiterated that laminectomy per se does not create sufficient instability to warrant the combined procedure of decompression and spinal fusion. Only demonstrable segmental or iatrogenic instability from bilateral foraminotomy at the same level is an indication for spinal fusion in addition to the decompression.

Indications for Fusion

The questions of what is the ideal surgical procedure and what is the role of spinal fusion in a degenerated intervertebral disc are as yet unanswered. When reviewing the literature in this field, one is reminded of Josh Billings' cryptic statement, "It ain't what a man don't know that makes him a fool but what he does know that ain't so." Semmes reviewed 1500 patients in whom only disc excision had been performed and found that 98 per cent considered themselves to have benefited from their operation.[11] At the other end of the spectrum, Young and Love reviewed a series of 450 patients with a combined procedure and 558 patients with disc excision alone and found that the combined operation relieved both symptoms in

20 per cent more patients than did the operation for removal of the disc alone and that there were three times as many failures to obtain relief of either back or leg pain when the fusion was not performed.[12] There are innumerable other follow-up studies in the literature that fail to resolve these questions. The answers will not be forthcoming until long-term prospective studies are undertaken in which patients in a definite diagnostic category are treated in a random and variable pattern. Until this is done, the proposed benefits of a considered spinal fusion will rest on less than solid ground.

At our present state of knowledge, spinal fusion should be undertaken for the following indications:

1. Acute disc herniations with a protracted significant component of back pain.

2. Chronic disc degeneration with significant back pain and degeneration limited to one or two disc levels.

3. Surgical instability created during decompression with bilateral removal of the facet joints.

4. The presence of neural arch defects coincident with disc disease.

5. The presence of symptomatic and radiographically demonstrable segmental instability.

SURGICAL TECHNIQUES

Simple Disc Excision

It must be emphasized that the procedure described subsequently is used in young people with evidence of acute, single level soft disc herniation in whom radicular symptoms predominate. This method is designed to minimize the postoperative recovery time yet effectively treat the source of nerve root compression, which is anticipated to be frankly herniated or extruded disc material.

ANESTHESIA

This operation may be performed under spinal, epidural, local, or general endotracheal anesthesia. The preference of the authors is the use of spinal anesthesia. The patient may be awake or asleep as he prefers, but in any event, the patient is able to breathe and cough for himself with minimal disturbance to his physiology. This policy has proved to be quite safe and satisfactory during the past ten years.

POSITION AT OPERATION

The patient is placed in a kneeling position, as described further on. The abdomen lies free, and the intra-abdominal pressure is reduced, thereby minimizing epidural venous bleeding. This position has proved to be of benefit, and since its adoption, epidural bleeding has virtually been eliminated as a cause for concern during surgery. When operative procedures were done in a prone position with pressure on the abdomen, the surgeon, not infrequently, could visualize distended epidural veins in the operative field. With the use of the abdomen-free kneeling position, however, the epidural veins are collapsed and offer little problem when encountered. Elastic stockings are used routinely.[13]

PREPARATION AND ANTIBIOTICS

Prophylactic antibiotics in the form of intravenous cefazolin sodium (Ancef) are utilized. A test dose of 0.5 gm. is administered the night prior to surgery to be certain that the patient has no allergy. The morning of surgery, the patient is given 0.5 gm. of Ancef intravenously; the second 0.5 gm. dose is given immediately before the incision is made. Intravenous Ancef is continued for 72 hours postoperatively at a dosage of 0.5 gm. IV every six hours. A wide area of the back is shaved and scrubbed with an antiseptic soap solution such as Betadine the night prior to surgery and again on the morning of surgery. Betadine solution is used for skin preparation in the operating room.

INCISION

Because this technique emphasizes performing a minimum of soft tissue dissection, accurate placement of the incision is required. Three criteria are utilized to place the incision, which is ordinarily 4 cm. long, directly over the affected disc:

1. Notation of the level of the iliac crest on the plain lumbar spine films.

2. Observation of the skin mark by the myelographic spinal puncture needle and correlation of this scar with the level of needle insertion on the myelographic studies.

3. Palpation of the last spinous process and the lumbosacral junction.

Using a combination of these landmarks, the surgeon can ordinarily satisfactorily locate the precise interspace of concern. The incision runs from the centers of the spinous processes of the vertebra between which the affected disc lies. Through this small incision, the paraspinous muscles are dissected free from the spinous process and the lamina on the appropriate side using subperiosteal dissection. The muscles are then held with a Taylor retractor. The point of the Taylor retractor is placed lateral to the facet joint and may be held either by an assistant or by a loop of roller gauze beneath the surgeon's foot. Meticulous hemostasis is obtained and all soft tissues are carefully curetted from the lamina above and below the involved interspace. The upper layers of the ligamentum flavum are also removed using a sharp curette so that accurate demonstration of the bony

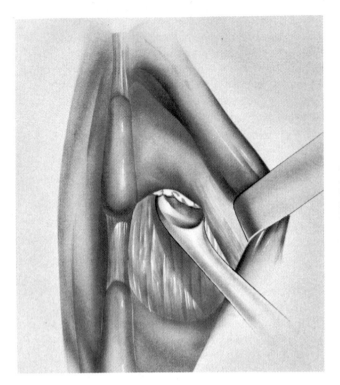

Figure 9–1. The posterior elements of the spine are cleaned of all soft tissue using sharp curettes. (From Rothman, R. H., and Simeone, F. A.: The Spine, 2nd ed. Philadelphia, W. B. Saunders Co., 1982.)

Figure 9–2. The limits of the ligamentum flavum are well defined as are the bony landmarks. (From Rothman, R. H., and Simeone, F. A.: The Spine, 2nd ed. Philadelphia, W. B. Saunders Co., 1982.)

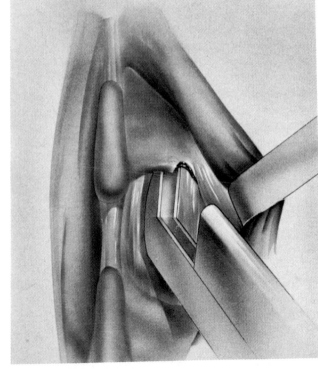

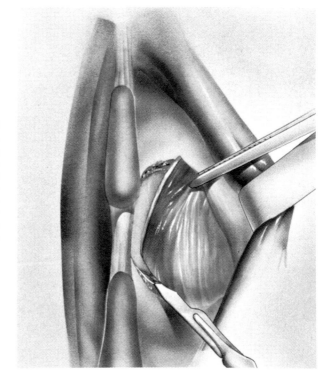

Figure 9–3. The extent of bone removal and ligamentum flavum removal prior to nerve root retraction. The lateral border of the nerve root is well seen before the nerve is retracted. Note the extruded nucleus beneath the nerve root. (From Rothman, R. H., and Simeone, F. A.: The Spine, 2nd ed. Philadelphia, W. B. Saunders Co., 1982.)

landmarks can be obtained and the level that is exposed can be rechecked (Fig. 9–1).

REMOVAL OF THE LIGAMENTUM FLAVUM

The ligamentum flavum beneath the superior lamina is separated utilizing a curette, and a small amount of bone is rongeured on the inferior margin of the superior lamina (Fig. 9–2). The limit of this bony resection is the free upper margin of the ligamentum flavum. At this point, magnifying loupes of two and one half power are applied, which greatly enhance the surgeon's ability to delineate fine structures.

The ligamentum flavum is opened with a #15 scalpel blade, and a long cottonoid pattie is inserted between the ligamentum flavum and the epidural tissue (Fig. 9–3). A long, thin cottonoid pattie is easily accepted in this space, thereby separating the dura from the subsequent dissection of the ligamentum flavum. The remaining ligament can be excised by sharp dissection or removed piecemeal with a Kerrison punch.

A modest amount of bone is now removed laterally and inferiorly until the surgeon is able to easily visualize the free lateral border of the nerve root (See Fig. 9–4). If the nerve root is distorted by the disc hernia or is anomalous, the surgeon will be unable to clearly define the lateral border of the root and further bone should be removed as necessary. This will circumvent the necessity of blindly inserting a root retractor and applying

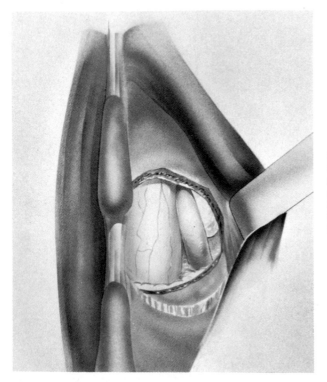

Figure 9–4. The ligamentum flavum is turned down with a fine forceps and excised using a small scalpel. The point of the knife is under direct vision. (From Rothman, R. H., and Simeone, F. A.: The Spine, 2nd ed. Philadelphia, W. B. Saunders Co., 1982.)

pressure to the delicate neural structures. Retraction should be undertaken only when the root is clearly defined.

NERVE ROOT INSPECTION

Once adequate bony resection is performed, the epidural fat surrounding the dura and nerve root may be gently removed with fine forceps and a Penfield dissector. The operator is now prepared to inspect the nerve root (Fig. 9–4). This is the most significant portion of the procedure because only by palpation and visualization can one assume that the appropriate nerve root is under pressure and thereby responsible for the radicular symptoms. Under loupe magnification, the nerve root is retracted medially with a Freer nasal septum elevator. A thinner instrument with a similar contour, the Penfield dissector, can separate the inferior surface of the nerve root from the floor of the spinal canal. When there is a significant disc herniation and particularly when there is a sequestered fragment, these two structures are frequently adherent. If difficulty is encountered in retraction of the nerve root, the operator can assume that there is pressure caused by bulging or extruded disc material. If frank extrusion is encountered at this point, an effort should be made to remove it fairly early in the dissection in order to avoid retraction injury to the nerve root. The extruded fragment should be removed intact, if possible, since portions of a fragmented nucleus may be difficult to find subsequently. If a protruding disc is encountered, as is frequently the case, 1 × 1 cm. cottonoid patties with radiopaque strings can be placed in the epidural space after the nerve root is gently retracted over the dome of the disc. These patties, placed above and below the disc herniation, can gently retract the nerve root and thereby enable one to avoid the hazards of a metal root retractor in the hands of an assistant. Ultimately, an area of the floor of the canal centered over the disc at least 1 cm. square should be visible. It may be necessary to extend the laminectomy laterally to obtain sufficient exposure. Removal of significant portions of the facet joint is occasionally necessary but has not caused significant symptomatology.

DISC EXCISION

A large rectangular window of the annulus is removed with a #15 knife blade on a long thin handle. This is often accompanied by spontaneous extrusion of the herniated nucleus. Straight and angled disc rongeurs are inserted into the nuclear material (Fig. 9–5). The surgeon should at all times be aware of the depth to which the rongeur is inserted. Although the jaws of the rongeur are operated by the right hand (for a right-handed surgeon), the left hand holds the shaft of the rongeur and prevents it from plunging when vigorous "bites" of disc material are extracted. The rongeur should never be closed until a sense of bone is felt against one of the end-plates. It must be re-emphasized that the jaws of the rongeur should

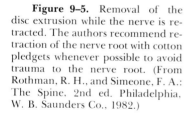

Figure 9–5. Removal of the disc extrusion while the nerve is retracted. The authors recommend retraction of the nerve root with cotton pledgets whenever possible to avoid trauma to the nerve root. (From Rothman, R. H., and Simeone, F. A.: The Spine, 2nd ed. Philadelphia, W. B. Saunders Co., 1982.)

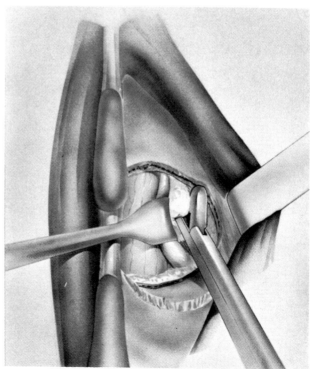

be in contact with the cartilaginous end-plates of the superior or inferior vertebra during the piecemeal removal of the disc material. This technique, along with the surgeon's undivided attention, will prevent plunging of the disc rongeur into the retroperitoneal space. When the central and lateral-most portions of the nucleus have been removed, the interspace is entered with a right-angled dural elevator, and the residual, more fibrotic disc material is separated from the annulus. It is forced into the center of the interspace and retrieved subsequently with disc rongeurs. Angled ring curettes are then inserted into the interspace, and the disc material is scraped from the cartilaginous end-plates and again retrieved. Care is taken to effect as complete an excision of disc material as is possible. A right-angled dural elevator is then placed between the nerve root and the site of the former disc herniation in the epidural space. Any residual bulging is flattened by forceful collapse of the elevated area into the interspace. This may force additional fragments of nuclear material into a position for subsequent removal.

At this point, a careful inspection of the epidural space about the nerve root is made with an appropriate instrument such as a Fraser elevator (Fig. 9–6). The nerve root should now be free of all compression and tension. If there is resistance to movement or tension, the procedure is not complete; a search must be made for extruded disc fragments, perhaps more remote from the laminectomy area in a cranial or caudal direction or lateral in the foramen.

If the nerve root appears to be compressed by the walls of the

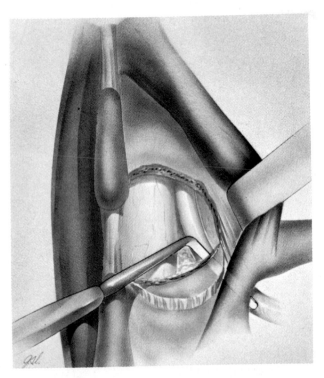

Figure 9–6. Exploration of the intervertebral foramen with a Fraser or malleable uterine probe. The nerve root should be free of both compression and tension. (From Rothman, R. H., and Simeone, F. A.: The Spine, 2nd ed. Philadelphia, W. B. Saunders Co., 1982.)

intervertebral foramen, a foraminotomy must be performed. With a Kerrison punch, bone is excised along the course of the exiting nerve root until all constriction is relieved. This may require partial or complete removal of the facet joint. Our experience indicates that significant portions of this joint can be excised at one level unilaterally without subsequent problems. Ultimately, the foraminotomy may extend well out beyond the confines of the spinal canal to the point at which the nerve root curves around the pedicle. If there is evidence of nerve root tension at this point, pedicle removal may be required.

At this point, the nerve root is usually quite free. It is not unusual, however, to expose 2 to 3 cm. of nerve root prior to effecting the desired "loose" feeling.

Once complete decompression of the root is accomplished, meticulous hemostasis is obtained using bipolar coagulation. Closing a wound over fleeting structures invites epidural hematoma and potential neurologic sequelae. Occasionally, five minutes of compression with Gelfoam and cottonoid patties will stop troublesome bleeding.

INTERPOSITION MEMBRANE

After the disc material has been radically removed and the nerve root is free, the entire exposed dura and root is covered with an autogenous fat graft. The graft is removed with scalpel dissections from the subcutaneous area, using great care not to interfere with the blood supply to the skin. If no fat is available, Gelfoam is utilized. The paraspinous muscles are approximated with 0 chromic suture, and the subcutaneous closure is made with 00 chromic suture. Wire staples are utilized for skin closure. The authors would use Hemovac drainage for even minor amounts of bleeding. The postoperative management is the same as described for the other laminectomy techniques described subsequently.

Lumbar Decompressive Laminectomy and Foraminotomy

This procedure is performed for most cases of symptomatic spinal stenosis, for large acute disc herniations with high-degree myelographic block, for multiple myelographic disc defects (particularly when the symptomatic disc is uncertain), and for situations of multiple nerve root involvement. The operation is designed to decompress the lumbar theca and appropriate nerve roots, especially when it may be impossible to actually remove the anteriorly placed source of compression.

ANESTHESIA

As with simple disc excisions, spinal anesthesia is the authors' method of choice.

POSITION AT OPERATION

The kneeling position, with abdomen free, is preferred (as previously described).

INCISION

The incision is made at midline and ordinarily spans the involved lower lumbar vertebrae. The fascia is incised throughout the length of the incision utilizing an electrocautery. With a broad, sharp periosteal elevator, the paraspinous muscles are dissected subperiosteally for the entire length of the incision. Frequent packing with dry sponges maintains hemostasis as the dissection continues. Large, self-retaining retractors are applied, and the appropriate spinous processes and the lamina and sacrum are identified. Meticulous hemostasis is maintained (Figs. 9–7 to 9–13).

Using the sharp-angled bone biter, the spinous processes of the appropriate laminae and the sacrum are removed. All soft tissue on and between the laminae is removed using large curettes, as are the upper layers of the ligamentum flavum. This allows for precise identification of the bony landmarks and the levels involved. The laminae are then removed, beginning with L5 and progressing in a cranial direction, using rongeurs of an appropriate size. Before using the rongeur, the ligamentum flavum is dissected free from the cranial margin of the lamina with a sharp

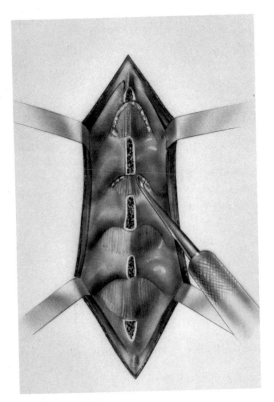

Figure 9–7. Preliminary step for performance of a lumbar decompressive laminectomy. Using sharp curettes, all soft tissues are removed from the lamina and interlaminar spaces down to the superficial layers of the ligamentum flavum. The curettes used must be sharp and ventral pressure must be avoided. Curettage should be performed against the bony surfaces. (From Rothman, R. H., and Simeone, F. A.: The Spine, 2nd ed. Philadelphia, W. B. Saunders Co., 1982.)

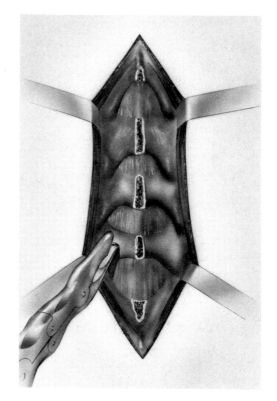

Figure 9–8. Removal of the lamina using a Lexcel rongeur. The rongeur jaws should be closed, then lifted in a ventral direction. Downward pressure must never be exerted against a compromised neural canal. (From Rothman, R. H., and Simeone, F. A.: The Spine, 2nd ed. Philadelphia, W. B. Saunders Co., 1982.)

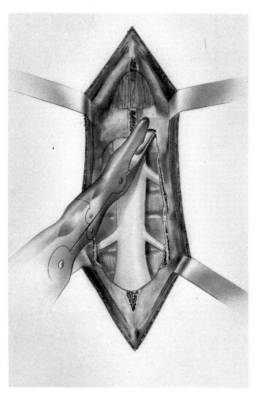

Figure 9–9. The lamina and ligamentum flavum are completely removed. The lateral portion of the facet joints are preserved if possible to retain the structural integrity and stability of the spine. With removal of the fifth, fourth, and a portion of the third lamina, the surgeon should be able to inspect the L4, L5, and S1 nerve roots bilaterally without difficulty. (From Rothman, R. H., and Simeone, F. A.: The Spine, 2nd ed. Philadelphia, W. B. Saunders Co., 1982.)

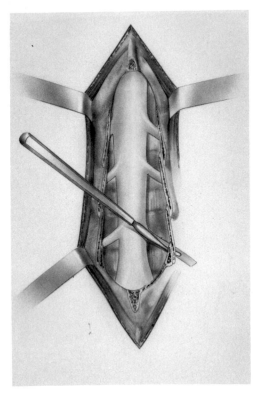

Figure 9–10. Each spinal nerve is followed into its foramen with a uterine probe or Fraser right-angled elevator to be certain that the root is under neither compression nor tension in the area of the lateral recess or foramen. (From Rothman, R. H., and Simeone, F. A.: The Spine, 2nd ed. Philadelphia, W. B. Saunders Co., 1982.)

Figure 9–11. Performance of a foraminotomy by removal of the dorsal portion of the facet joints with an angled Schlessinger punch. The instruments follow the path of the spinal nerve with great caution never to exert ventral compression on the neural elements. If the Schlessinger punch will not fit in the foramen, a Sella punch or air drill can be utilized. (From Rothman, R. H., and Simeone, F. A.: The Spine, 2nd ed. Philadelphia, W. B. Saunders Co., 1982.)

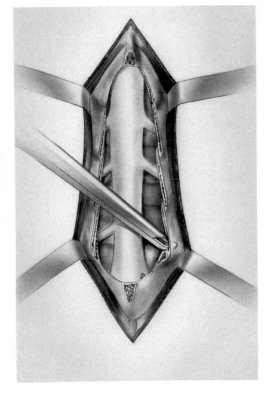

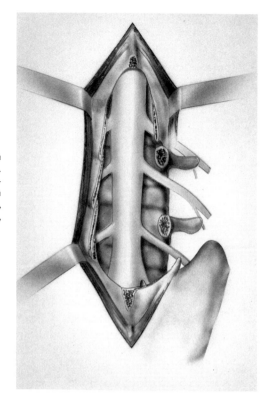

Figure 9–12. Complete foraminotomy on the right, unroofing the L4 and L5 spinal nerves. The lateral portion of the facet joints are preserved on the left to avoid spinal instability. (From Rothman, R. H., and Simeone, F. A.: The Spine, 2nd ed. Philadelphia, W. B. Saunders Co., 1982.)

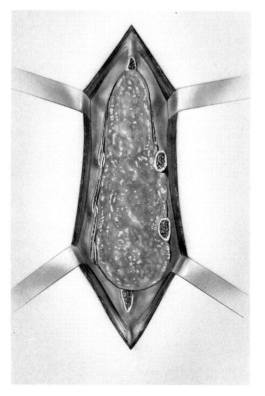

Figure 9–13. At the conclusion of the decompression, an autogenous fat graft is placed about the exposed surface of the dura and spinal nerve to prevent scar tissue formation. (From Rothman, R. H., and Simeone, F. A.: The Spine, 2nd ed. Philadelphia, W. B. Saunders Co., 1982.)

curette. The L5 lamina is removed first because the spatial relations allow the easiest access to this level. In the usual case of spinal stenosis, L3 to L4 and L4 to L5 are more frequently collapsed and shingled, making the L5 lamina most readily accessible for the initial stages of the decompression.

When there is evidence of marked neural compression, the procedure must be done carefully with small rongeurs. Ultimately, the appropriate laminae are removed laterally to the medial surface of the pedicles.

Once the laminae have been excised, residual ligamentum flavum is removed using a scalpel or a Kerrison punch. The nerve roots are then inspected for tension and compression. Almost without exception, we will inspect the L4, L5, and S1 nerve roots on the involved side. In most instances, the surgeon encounters only a diffuse bulging annulus in spinal stenosis, but occasionally, a coincident disc herniation is also found.

Only when a true herniation is present do we enter the disc space and attempt to remove nuclear material. In the usual case of spinal stenosis, a dorsal decompression will completely eliminate nerve root compression.

If compression of the nerve root is noted in the lateral recesses beneath the facet joint or further laterally in the foramen, decompression of the lateral recess or foraminotomy is performed. Angled Kerrison punches are used to perform this lateral decompression, following the course of the nerve root until alleviation of all compression is attained.

Occasionally, a foramen will be so tightly compressed that even a small cervical punch cannot be inserted without traumatizing the nerve root. In these unusual situations, a Hall drill can be utilized to remove bone until only a thin shell remains over the nerve root. This thin shell is then removed with a fine-angled curette. As the foraminotomy proceeds, it is prudent to be certain that there are no free fragments of disc material that have migrated laterally into the foramen.

Depending on the pathologic condition found, foraminotomy will be performed at all necessary levels on the symptomatic side. In most instances, the sciatica is unilateral, and foraminotomy need not be performed on the asymptomatic side. We attempt to maintain the integrity of the facet joints on the asymptomatic side whenever possible and do not perform extensive explorations of asymptomatic nerve roots. However, if bilateral foraminotomies must be performed, the decompression is ordinarily followed by a lateral spine fusion of the unstable segments.

WOUND CLOSURE

The paraspinous muscles are approximated with 0 chromic suture and the subcutaneous tissues closed with 00 chromic gut. The skin is closed with staples. If meticulous hemostasis is maintained, closed drainage is not necessary. However, if there is the least doubt as to hemostasis, the authors would use Hemovac drainage. Postoperative management is similar to that indicated for the fusion procedure (see further on).

INTERPOSITION MEMBRANE

Scar formation about the dural sac and nerve roots after surgical intervention constitutes one of the most frequent causes of postoperative pain. In our experience, scar formation is almost always present to a greater or lesser extent. It acts as a constrictive force about the neural elements and also tethers the nerve roots to the spine. For reasons that are not well explained, the scar formation causes symptomatology in certain patients and not in others. It may be present for several months or a year before the symptoms become apparent. Surgical removal of the scar tissue in the past has usually led to its recurrence in a short time. Thus, it was with great interest that surgeons concerned with the spine greeted the research of MacNab[14] on the etiology and prevention of postoperative scar formation in the neural canal. In the experimental animal, McNab clearly showed the relationship of postoperative dural scarring to surgically exposed muscle. This tendency toward scar formation could be markedly inhibited by the interposition of a resorbable Gelfoam membrane. Attention to atraumatic technique and complete hemostasis are also of obvious importance.

No clinical reports are as yet available on the use of Gelfoam membranes. The authors have used this type of Gelfoam membrane about all areas of the dura and nerve roots for a period of four years in over 300 cases of nerve root decompression. No ill effects have become evident, although the period of follow-up evaluation is as yet too short to make a general conclusion.

More recently, the authors have used an autogenous fat graft, where available, rather than Gelfoam membranes. This is based on the laboratory studies of Langenskiöld, Gill, and Jacobs that have indicated that autogenous fat is a more effective deterrent to scar tissue formation than Gelfoam.[15, 16, 17] Where fat is not available, Gelfoam continues to be utilized.

Lateral Spine Fusion

When arthrodesis of the spine is necessary, the authors currently recommend the use of bilateral lateral fusion. Many variations of this technique have been reported in the past.[18, 19, 20] There are several advantages in the use of a lateral fusion. Foremost among these are the certainty

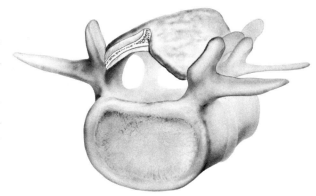

Figure 9–14. This drawing illustrates iatrogenic spinal stenosis due to a midline spinal fusion. The decortication of lamina and application of bone graft in the midline created spinal stenosis through two mechanisms. The first of these is thickening of the lamina and the second is overgrowth of the fusion mass at the cranial end of the fusion dipping into the interspace and compressing the neural elements. (From Rothman, R. H., and Simeone, F. A.: The Spine, 2nd ed. Philadelphia, W. B. Saunders Co., 1982.)

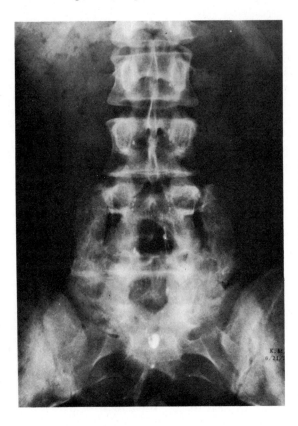

Figure 9–15. Well formed bilateral lateral spinal fusion from L4 to the sacrum. Note the massive appearance of the bone graft from the transverse process of L4 to the ala of the sacrum. No graft material is placed in the midline. (From Rothman, R. H., and Simeone, F. A.: The Spine, 2nd ed. Philadelphia, W. B. Saunders Co., 1982.)

of obtaining a solid fusion, the ability to perform the fusion in the absence of posterior elements, and the prevention of iatrogenic spinal stenosis (Figs. 9–14, 9–15).

ANESTHESIA

This operation is performed under spinal anesthesia. Cardiac monitors are used for elderly individuals and for patients with a history of cardiovascular disease.

POSITION AT OPERATION

The procedure is performed in the prone position. If decompressive laminectomy or disc excision is to be performed at the same time, the kneeling position is utilized to ensure collapse of the epidural veins and to minimize abdominal compression (Fig. 9–16). If only a spinal fusion is to be performed, the patient is placed on a flat operating table with lateral rolls beneath the chest and abdomen to allow breathing space. The anterior iliac crest is centered over the kidney rest, permitting flexion of the table if desired to reduce the lumbar lordosis. The patient wears elastic stockings to prevent thrombophlebitis.

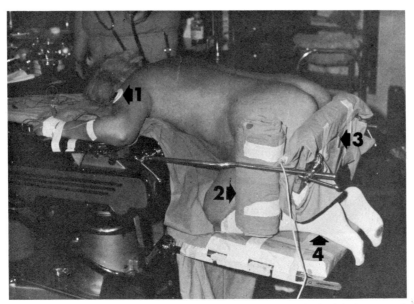

Figure 9–16. Kneeling position utilized for laminectomy and spinal fusion. Note how, even in this obese patient, the abdomen is completely free preventing any pressure on the vena cava.

    1. EKG monitoring is used because of the difficulty of listening to the heart sounds in this position.

    2. Lateral padding is used to stabilize the patient and prevent pressure on the side bars.

    3. The patient is stabilized caudally by the use of a seat to prevent extreme flexion at the knees and hips.

    4. Elastic stockings or elastic bandages are used to prevent pooling of blood in the calf area.

(From Rothman, R. M., and Simeone, F. A.: The Spine, 2nd ed. Philadelphia, W. B. Saunders Co., 1982.)

ANTIBIOTICS

The use of prophylactic antibiotics is advised, as outlined previously.

INCISION

A hockey stick incision is utilized, with the lower pole deviating to the side where the iliac crest graft will be obtained. If an L4 to the sacrum fusion is to be performed, the incision starts above the third lumbar spinous process, continues in a caudal direction to the sacral spinous process, and then deviates gradually two inches in a lateral direction (Fig. 9–17). The horizontal component of the lower end of the incision allows easy access to the ilium to obtain graft material. The vertical limb of the incision is carried directly down to the fascia in the midline, without the creation of layers. Absolute hemostasis is obtained at this step. Then, utilizing the electric cutting knife, the fascia is incised from above the third spinous process to the lower portion of the sacrum. Subsequently, utilizing a broad sharp periosteal elevator, the paraspinal muscles are stripped subperiosteally from the spine. This dissection is carried to the facet joints. As the dissection progresses, the wound is packed tightly with sponges to

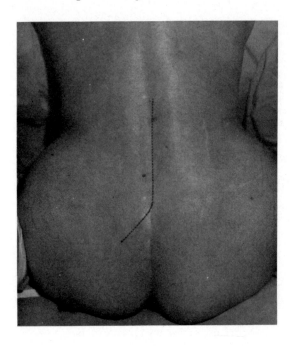

Figure 9–17. Hockey stick incision used for a two level spinal fusion from L4 to the sacrum. Incision extends from the third lumbar spinous process to the sacrum and then deviates laterally to allow exposure of the iliac crest. (From Rothman, R. H., and Simeone, F. A.: The Spine, 2nd ed. Philadelphia, W. B. Saunders Co., 1982.)

control bleeding. When this is completed, the sponges are removed, and large self-retaining retractors are placed to expose the posterior elements of the spine. At this point, the surgeon should orient himself carefully through the sacrum and the lower lumbar vertebrae to be certain he is working at the correct levels.

Utilizing a large, sharp-angled bone biter, the spinous processes of the sacrum, the fourth and fifth lumbar vertebrae, and a portion of the third spinous process are removed. The soft tissues are then meticulously dissected and removed from the posterior elements of the spine down to the ligamentum flavum. This is accomplished with large sharp curettes. The dissection is most easily accomplished when started laterally at the facet joints and when the tissues are swept toward the midline, where they are removed with the scalpel. The correct use of the curette is mandatory. Pressure should never be exerted in a downward direction. Rather, the curette should be directed cranially or caudally, allowing it to cut the soft tissues cleanly from bone. It should be stressed that a large curette is infinitely safer than a small one in this area.

If nerve root exploration and decompression are to be undertaken they may start at this juncture. If not, attention is turned to exposure of the transverse processes. Using either the electric knife or a sharp periosteal elevator, the fascia is incised directly laterally to the facet joints of L3–L4. As this fascia is incised, the periosteal elevator can sweep laterally along the superior articular facet of L4 and down onto the fourth transverse process. Paraspinal muscles can then be swept laterally, exposing the entire length of the transverse process. When the process is cleaned of soft tissue and completely exposed on its dorsal aspect, the area should be packed with a sponge to control bleeding. The incision in the fascia should then be continued in a caudal direction and, utilizing the L4–L5 facet joint as a landmark, the fifth transverse process should be exposed in a similar manner. All ligaments and muscles should be dissected well laterally, forming an uninterrupted gutter between the transverse processes and the ala of the sacrum. After the fifth transverse process is exposed, cleaned, and packed, the fascia incision is continued down to a point distal and lateral to the superior articular facet of the sacrum. Dissection lateral to this element will expose the ala of the sacrum. Many dense ligaments are adherent in this area and must be dissected from the sacrum in order to clearly expose the ala. It is essential to clearly visualize both the transverse processes and the ala in order to obtain an optimal preparation of the fusion bed. The sponges previously used to obtain hemostasis about the transverse processes and the ala of the sacrum are then removed, and a careful decortication of the transverse processes, the lateral portion of the pedicles, and the lateral portion of the articular facets is performed. This is best accomplished with large, sharp curettes. Some care is required in order not to fracture the transverse process.

The ala of the sacrum is best decorticated with a narrow, round gouge. The lateral portion of the superior articular facet of the sacrum should also be decorticated. A hole is created in the cranial portion of the ala of the sacrum using a large curette, which will ultimately receive a portion of the graft material. This process of exposure and decortication is repeated on both sides of the spine. The wound is again carefully packed, and the midline fascia is closed with a towel clip.

BONE GRAFT

The posterior iliac crest is exposed by dissecting away the layer of adipose tissue with a large sponge. The fascia is incised in line with the posterior iliac crest and the crest is then dissected subperiosteally. The gluteal muscles are carefully dissected from the lateral wing of the ilium. Care must be taken to remain beneath the periosteum, or dramatic bleeding that is difficult to control can occur. A broad reverse retractor is then inserted to clearly expose the lateral position of the ilium. Utilizing sharp, curved gouges, long strips of cortical and cancellous bone are removed from the ilium until the inner wall of the ilium is exposed. Large amounts of bone are readily obtained from this area. This graft material should be cut into strips approximately 1 to 2 mm. in width and saved in blood-soaked sponges (Fig. 9–18).

PLACEMENT OF THE GRAFT MATERIAL AND CLOSURE OF THE WOUND

The midline wound is then re-exposed and the self-retaining retractors are reinserted. All the sponges are removed from the wound, and the wound is checked with careful finger palpation to be certain that none of the recesses harbor a hidden sponge. At this point, the preliminary sponge count should be obtained. The graft material is then placed in the trough that has been created from the fourth transverse process to the ala of the sacrum bilaterally (Fig. 9–19).

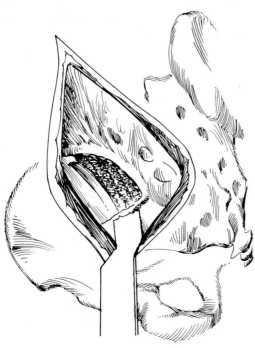

Figure 9–18. Technique of obtaining autogenous graft material from the posterior iliac crest. A large spiked retractor is utilized to expose the posterior surface of the ilium. Long strips of cortical and cancellous bone are then obtained, utilizing curved gouges. The graft material is saved in blood-soaked sponges and transferred to the previously prepared bed within five minutes. (From Rothman, R. H., and Simeone, F. A.: The Spine, 2nd ed. Philadelphia, W. B. Saunders Co., 1982.)

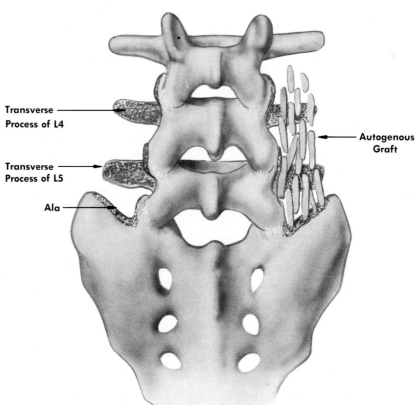

Transverse Process of L4

Transverse Process of L5

Ala

Autogenous Graft

Figure 9–19. Area of the bed of raw cancellous bone for a lateral spine fusion from L4 to the sacrum. The bed is shown on the left and the graft material is in place on the right. In actuality a much larger volume of graft material is utilized. The bed includes the transverse processes, the ala of the sacrum, the lateral portion of the pedicle and the lateral portion of the superior articular facets. (From Rothman, R. H., and Simeone, F. A.: The Spine, 2nd ed. Philadelphia, W. B. Saunders Co., 1982.)

The wounds should be frequently irrigated with antibiotic solution, and, at this point, all devitalized tissue should be debrided. The double-limb suction drain is inserted with one limb deep in the midline wound and the other at the iliac crest donor site. The fascia is then closed using #1 chromic suture. Subcutaneous closure is obtained with 00 chromic suture, and the skin edges are approximated with metallic staples.

POSTOPERATIVE MANAGEMENT

The patient is allowed out of bed and may walk the day after surgery. If there is difficulty in voiding, the patient may be permitted to stand at his bedside on the night of surgery. This may circumvent the need for catheterization with its attendant risk of infection. An exercise program is started on the second or third postoperative day, with deep knee bends and tuck exercises with the knees being drawn to the chest. No external supports such as braces or corsets are used. This program of early mobilization has not been shown to lower the rate of successful fusion and has many dramatic advantages. Psychologically, the patient becomes attuned to an optimistic course and early return to productive life. The paraspinal muscles rapidly resume their normal tone, and the resolution of edema and hematoma occurs quickly.

The suction drains are withdrawn and the dressings removed at 48 hours. The wound remains exposed to the air after this point. It is sprayed with Betadine (povidone-iodine) twice daily. Narcotics or mild analgesics are utilized for the first few postoperative days as needed. Antibiotics, as previously noted, are administered for 72 hours postoperatively. The staples are removed and the patient is discharged in ten days.

Subsequent to discharge, the patient is encouraged to gradually increase his level of activity. He is advised that the pain in his spine should be the guideline to his level of activity and that this should not be exceeded. Automobile riding is prohibited for the first several weeks. Heavy lifting is also discouraged. After four to six weeks, the patient may return to light work, at least on a part-time basis. After three months, most patients are able to return full time to sedentary and moderately active employment. Heavy physical labor is prohibited for six months. The same is true of vigorous athletics.

The patient is reevaluated at six-week intervals for the first three months and then at three-month intervals for the first year. As recovery progresses, the patient is placed on a more vigorous program of flexion exercises and is again instructed as to the essential aspects of back hygiene. He is encouraged to return to a normal way of life as rapidly as possible.

Anterior Interbody Fusion

This type of fusion should be reserved for certain patients who have had multiple surgical procedures through the posterior approach to the spine that have failed. Dense posterior scarring, wide resection of the posterior elements of the spine, and a failed lateral spinal fusion are indications for consideration of this technique. The major disadvantage inherent in this surgical approach is the inability to carefully explore and decompress nerve roots when this is required.

This operation should be performed by a spinal surgeon and an abdominal surgeon together, unless the spinal surgeon has had extensive experience with the anterior approach.

ANESTHESIA

A nasogastric tube is utilized to prevent abdominal distention. Endotracheal anesthesia is preferred with the patient in the Trendelenburg position.

APPROACH

The retroperitoneal approach described by Harmon is utilized. A left paramedian incision is made, the anterior rectus sheath is opened, and the muscle is retracted laterally. The retroperitoneal space is entered, and the peritoneum is dissected bluntly from the undersurface of the posterior rectus sheath.[21] The peritoneum is mobilized, and as the lower lumbar spine is exposed, the ureter is left in its peritoneal bed and reflected to the right. The sacral promontory is identified by palpation. It is essential not to damage the sympathetic nerves coursing over the sacrum. The major sympathetic chains on either side of the lumbar vertebrae are carefully dissected and retracted in a lateral direction. The L5 interspace is exposed by retracting the left iliac artery and vein to the left and the right iliac artery and vein to the right. To expose the fourth lumbar vertebra, the left artery and vein are displaced to the right side of the spine. Spiked retractors are driven into the body of the vertebra to maintain exposure.

ANTERIOR DISC EXCISION AND FUSION

The anterior longitudinal ligament is elevated as a flap, with the base attached on the left. Exposure can be improved at this time by hyperextension of the operating table and spine. Then, utilizing the sharp osteotome, curettes, and rongeurs, the entire disc is excised and a trough created in the opposing surfaces of the vertebral body above and below. The dimensions of this space are then measured, and three cortical-cancellous grafts are obtained from the left iliac crest. The grafts should be slightly larger than the notch so that firm impaction can be obtained. After insertion of the three grafts, the spine can be brought to a neutral position, locking the grafts in place (Fig. 9–20). The previously created flap of anterior longitudinal ligament can be reattached or, if this is not possible, excised. The wound is closed in a routine manner after hemostasis is obtained. An excellent comprehensive discussion of the role, techniques,

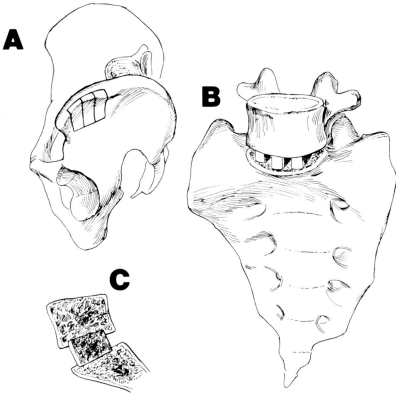

Figure 9–20. Technique of anterior lumbar fusion. After excision of the intervertebral disc, cortical cancellous grafts from the iliac crest are inserted into countersunk panels created in the adjacent vertebral end plates. (From Rothman, R. H., and Simeone, F. A.: The Spine, 2nd ed. Philadelphia, W. B. Saunders Co., 1982.)

and results of anterior disc excision and fusion was presented by Goldner.[22]

POSTOPERATIVE MANAGEMENT

The nasogastric tube is removed after peristalsis returns. Elastic stockings, early ambulation, and prophylactic anticoagulation are utilized to prevent thrombophlebitis. The management in other respects is similar to that after lateral spine fusion.

RESULTS OF OPERATIVE TREATMENT OF LUMBAR DISC DISEASE

Over three decades have passed since the advent of surgical treatment of lumbar disc disease. Improvement in the efficiency of surgical treatment must be predicated on accurate knowledge of the quality of result that can be expected with each technique and diagnosis. Long-term follow-up is

TABLE 9–1. Population*

Mean age surgery	40 years
Mean age follow up	48 years
Mean follow up	8 years
Range follow up	1–20 years
Ten year or greater follow up	195 patients

*From Rothman, R. H., and Simeone, F. A.: The Spine, 2nd ed. Philadelphia, W. B. Saunders Co., 1982.

essential in this area, and studies of this type are available in the literature. The pressing need at the present time is for an accurately constructed prospective study using various surgical techniques for each of the specific diagnostic entities under consideration. Retrospective studies grouping all disc diseases into one diagnostic category are of limited value.

DePalma and Rothman have reported their experience over a period of 20 years with over 1500 patients who had undergone surgery for lumbar disc degeneration.[23] These patients were called back for personal interview, physical examination, and repeat radiographic examination, including stress films. In order to minimize bias, the evaluations were performed by physicians other than the operating surgeon.

Examination of the population distribution curve revealed that the average age at surgery was 40, with a normal frequency distribution above and below this level. This age distribution is in keeping with the more recent pathologic concepts of disc degeneration. The average age of follow-up evaluation was 48, and the average follow-up period was eight years. One hundred and ninety-five patients were followed for a period of 10 years or longer (Table 9–1).

Relief of symptoms was the most important criterion for success in terms of low back surgery. Patients were questioned about the degree and temporal nature of their relief of back and leg pain. Their evaluation as to the subjective worth of their surgery was also elicited.

In individuals with L5 disc degeneration, 15 per cent had persistent back pain, 7 per cent had persistent sciatica, and 14 per cent had both back

TABLE 9–2. Percentages of Disc Degeneration Patients Showing Symptoms at Follow Up*

	L5–S1	L4–L5	Both
Preoperative			
Back pain	10	7	7
Leg pain	5	0	4
Both	85	93	89
Postoperative			
Back pain	15	17	11
Leg pain	7	7	4
Both	14	17	20

*From Rothman, R. H., and Simeone, F. A.: The Spine, 2nd ed. Philadelphia, W. B. Saunders Co., 1982.

TABLE 9–3. Patients With Disc Degeneration
Showing Subjective Relief at Follow Up*

	L5–S1	L4–L5	Both
Total	62	67	59
Partial	30	24	28
Temporary	4	7	11
None	3	3	2
Surgery worthwhile	88	88	75

*From Rothman, R. H., and Simeone, F. A.: The
Spine, 2nd ed. Philadelphia, W. B. Saunders Co., 1982.

pain and sciatica. The results are approximately the same with L4 disc
degeneration and two-level disc degeneration (Table 9–2). When questioned as to overall relief of their pain, approximately 60 per cent of
individuals in each category stated that they had obtained complete relief
of back and leg pain, approximately 30 per cent considered themselves
partially relieved, and 2 to 3 per cent were a total failure with no relief
whatsoever. Of the patients with disc degeneration at L4 or L5, 88 per cent
felt their surgery worthwhile; the percentage was less when both disc
spaces were affected (Table 9–3).

Physical findings were evaluated at follow up and compared to preoperative findings. The nonspecific findings such as muscle spasm, tenderness, and limitation of motion and straight leg raising disappeared in 90
per cent of those individuals who showed these findings preoperatively.
Neurologic deficits returned to normal less often postoperatively. Motor
and sensory deficits that had been present preoperatively disappeared in
50 per cent of the patients. Only 25 per cent of the patients lost their
preoperative reflex changes. This is somewhat better than the results
reported by Knutsson, in which only 33 per cent of patients lost their
sensory deficit, 24 per cent lost their motor deficit and 2½ per cent lost
their reflex abnormalities[24] (Table 9–4).

Certain general observations were noted that are also of interest. An
attempt was made to select those factors that would be of poor prognostic
significance for the patient undergoing back surgery.

In regard to diagnosis, high discs (i.e., above the L4–L5 level) did more

TABLE 9–4. Percentage Changes in Physical
Findings After Surgery*

Loss of all reflex change	25
Loss of all motor deficit	50
Loss of all sensory deficit	50
Loss of abnormal curve	
Muscle spasm	
Tenderness	90 or
Limited motion	more
Straight leg raising	

*From Rothman, R. H., and Simeone, F. A.: The
Spine, 2nd ed. Philadelphia, W. B. Saunders Co., 1982.

TABLE 9–5. Percentage of Patients Who Considered Surgery Worthwhile*

Pseudarthrosis	Solid Fusion
82	92

*From Rothman, R. H., and Simeone, F. A.: The Spine, 2nd ed. Philadelphia, W. B. Saunders Co., 1982.

poorly in regard to relief of symptomatology. One operative category appeared to fare more poorly — lumbosacral fusion combined with disc excision alone at the L4–L5 level. At one time, this operation was felt to be appropriate when a degenerated L4–L5 disc was found together with evidence of an unstable lumbosacral mechanism. The correlation of physical findings with quality of result revealed that a negative straight leg raising test in the preoperative examination tended to correspond with a poor result. This observation was also noted by Hirsch.[25] He determined that laminectomy and exploration were negative more often when the straight leg raising test, neurologic examination, and myelogram were negative. He further observed that with negative exploration the quality of result was poor regardless of the operative procedure performed.

Pseudarthrosis

The overall rate of solid fusion in the above series was 92 per cent, with an 8 per cent incidence of pseudarthrosis. Following the advent of the lateral fusion technique, the incidence of pseudarthrosis in two-level fusions is 6 per cent.[26] The incidence of pseudarthrosis in one-level fusions utilizing the lateral technique is less than 1 per cent. In our study group, 39 patients were discovered whom we could classify radiographically as having definite pseudarthrosis. In the hope of learning in detail what the diagnosis of pseudarthrosis portends for a patient, we studied these individuals in detail. They were compared with a matched group of 39 patients, each having an identical diagnosis and operation in whom the fusion was solid. By comparing these two matched groups, we can state with some degree of precision the implication of pseudarthrosis for the patient who has undergone a spinal fusion.

TABLE 9–6. Percentage of Patients Receiving Relief From Symptoms*

	Pseudarthrosis	Solid Fusion
Total	56	61
Partial	34	26
Temporary	10	5
None	0	8

*From Rothman, R. H., and Simeone, F. A.: The Spine, 2nd ed. Philadelphia, W. B. Saunders Co., 1982.

**TABLE 9–7.   Percentages of Patients
With Back Pain at Follow Up***

	Pseudarthrosis	Solid Fusion
Preoperative	92	97
Postoperative	44	38

*From Rothman, R. H., and Simeone, F. A.: The
Spine, 2nd ed. Philadelphia, W. B. Saunders Co., 1982.

In an overall subjective evaluation of the worth of their surgery, 82 per
cent of the patients who had developed pseudarthrosis felt that their
surgery was worthwhile, whereas 92 per cent of the group who had solid
fusions felt that their surgery was worthwhile (Table 9–5). Little difference
was found between the pseudoarthrosis group and the solid fusion group
when they were asked specifically about their overall relief from symptomatology. Fifty-six per cent of patients in the former group and 61 per cent
in the latter group obtained total relief. It is interesting to note that,
although there was a slight decrease in the number who obtained total
relief in the pseudarthrosis group, three patients who achieved solid
fusions obtained no relief, and all patients who developed pseudarthrosis
obtained at least partial or temporary relief (Table 9–6).

When back pain alone was considered, of the 92 per cent of patients in
the pseudarthrosis group who originally had back pain, 44 per cent still
had the symptoms at follow-up evaluation. In the solid fusion group, of the
97 per cent of patients who originally had back pain, 38 per cent had
significant back pain at follow-up evaluation (Table 9–7).

Sciatica was eliminated more consistently than back pain at follow-up
evaluation. Of the 79 per cent of patients in the pseudarthrosis group who
had sciatica, only 25 per cent had their symptoms at follow-up evaluation.
In the solid-fusion group, of the 85 per cent of patients who originally had
sciatica, only 20 per cent had their symptoms at follow-up evaluation
(Table 9–8). The subjective factors noted above were submitted to Chi-
square analysis and in no case was a significant difference noted between
the pseudarthrosis group and the solid fusion group. It seems justifiable to
draw certain conclusions from the preceding information. One of two
situations must exist: either the pseudarthrosis represents a fibrous stabilization that is essentially as effective as bony fusion, or the fusion component of these procedures was not essential. The former is not unreason-
able, as the amount of motion demonstrated on flexion-extension films of

**TABLE 9–8.   Percentage of Patients
With Sciatica at Follow Up***

	Pseudarthrosis	Solid Fusion
Preoperative	79	85
Postoperative	25	20

*From Rothman, R. H., and Simeone, F. A.: The
Spine, 2nd ed. Philadelphia, W. B. Saunders Co., 1982.

pseudarthrosis is usually minimal and is often less than 2 ml. The latter conclusion, however, remains in question.

Furthermore, it would seem prudent to carefully observe patients with pseudarthrosis for a rather prolonged period of time before reoperating in an attempt to achieve union. There seems to be little rationale for submitting patients to multiple attempts at repair of pseudarthrosis if, as a group, there is little difference in their subjective result when solid fusion is obtained.

The overall picture that develops is that a certain number of patients who have undergone spinal fusion continue to have back pain and less frequently sciatica, whether or not their fusion has become solid. The success rate, as judged by objective evaluation, is slightly greater in that group that has achieved solid fusion. Pseudarthrosis, of itself, does not appear to be the dreaded complication that is often portrayed. A more precise definition of the role of spinal fusion and evaluation of the essentiality of achieving this fusion will depend on the availability of long term prospective studies of spinal surgery.

As one reviews the overwhelming amount of written material pertaining to spinal surgery, certain precepts become clear and certain requirements evident, if good results are to be obtained.

Requirements for Successful Spinal Surgery

1. Accurate knowledge of the variable pathology of disc degeneration.
2. Accurate diagnosis of nerve root compression.
3. Adherence to the proper criterion for surgical intervention.
4. Selection of the proper operative procedure.
5. Skillful execution of the surgical procedure by an experienced spinal surgeon.
6. The prompt recognition and treatment of complications.
7. Careful postoperative care and rehabilitation.

If every patient undergoing spine surgery had the benefit of these principles, the quality of surgical result would improve dramatically, and the grey veil of apprehension, fear, and anxiety that has surrounded spinal surgery for years would be lifted.

COMPLICATIONS OF LUMBAR DISC SURGERY

The basic precept of all surgeons is, "above all, do no harm." The prevention of complications in spine surgery demands an awareness of all the potential hazards, a thorough knowledge of standard and variational anatomy, and meticulous surgical technique. Despite elaborate precautions and great care, however, these complications may occur but should be recognized early and treated appropriately.

Complications During Operation

VASCULAR AND VISCERAL INJURIES

Injuries to the great vessels, including the aorta, inferior vena cava, and iliac vessels, as well as other visceral structures, occur from penetration of the inferior portion of the annulus with surgical instruments. These injuries can carry serious implications with a mortality of up to 78 per cent if the injury is arterial and up to 89 per cent if the injury is venous.[34]

The majority of these injuries occur while trying to clean the anterior portion of the disc space with a curette or pituitary rongeur. An erroneous estimation of the depth of the interspace will lead to penetration of the annulus by the instrument and traumatization of one of the large vessels. It is important to remember that the anterior annulus does not necessarily have to be violated by surgical instruments, since the degenerative disc process affects not only the posterior aspect of the annulus but the anterior aspect as well.[44]

The aorta and vena cava lie in approximation to the L4 disc space, whereas the iliac vessels lie in approximation to the L5 disc space (Fig. 9–21).[46]

Immediate laceration that violates the lumen of these vessels may occur with massive hemorrhage; partial injuries to the wall of a vessel with delayed hemorrhage may occur or there can be laceration of both an artery and vein with a resultant arteriovenous fistula.

There tends to be a delay in the diagnosis of arteriovenous fistula following discectomy, primarily since in the majority of cases reported, no bleeding was appreciated from the disc space at the time of surgery.[40] This unique complication occurs more often at the L4–L5 interspace because of the proximity of the iliac artery and vein. The right common iliac artery has been most susceptible to injury, with venous injuries equally distributed among the left and right iliac veins and the inferior vena cava. Approximately half of the cases reported were diagnosed within one month of surgery, and 70 per cent were diagnosed within six months. A majority of

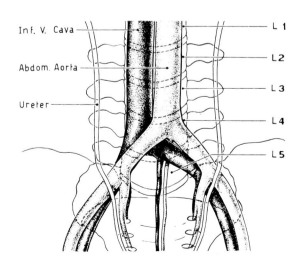

Figure 9–21. Relationship between the great vessels and the lumbar disc spaces. (From Montorsi, W., and Ghiringhelli, C.: Genesis, diagnosis, and treatment of vascular complications after intervertebral disc surgery. Int. Surg. *58*:233, 1973.)

patients presented with signs and symptoms of high output cardiac decompensation, specifically tachycardia with or without cardiomegaly, orthopnea caused by congestive heart failure, and a to-and-fro machinery-type lower abdominal bruit.[40] Injury to the ureter[47] and the appendix[30] have also been reported and have been associated with arteriovenous fistulas. Fortunately, despite the delay in diagnoses and treatment, a comparatively low mortality of only approximately 8 per cent has been reported.

Prevention of these injuries will be enhanced if adequate exposure is undertaken during surgery. If adequate exposure and hemostasis are not obtained prior to entering the disc space, continuous epidural bleeding will obscure the field of vision and will make it difficult to estimate the depth of the disc space. The depth with which an instrument penetrates the disc space should never exceed 1⅛ inches. The surgeon who occasionally performs spine surgery should have the instruments marked in this regard. Even skilled surgeons, however, must constantly keep this dimension in mind while working in the depths of the disc space. A third and most important precaution is that every instrument tip should be against bone while cleaning a disc space. Pituitary rongeurs should not be closed unless the rasp of metal upon bone is felt, nor should the stroke of a curette be continued unless this reassuring sensation is felt.

Further avoidance of these dreaded complications is provided by the patient being placed in the kneeling or tucked position used by the authors, since it decreases epidural pressure and subsequently affords better exposure of the disc space; also importantly, the abdominal contents, including the major vessels, will tend to drift ventrally away from the spine during the course of surgery.

Awareness of the possibility of this complication is important, and prompt surgical intervention is the only effective treatment. Profuse bleeding from the disc space or hypovolemic shock disproportionate to the observable blood loss should alert the surgeon to the potentiality. The management of the complication is immediate laparotomy and repair of the vascular injury. The spinal wound should be closed immediately with towel clips and a sterile plastic drape. Blood and fluid replacement should begin immediately, and the patient should be turned to the supine position while a vascular surgeon is summoned.

AIR EMBOLISM

Although very rare, the kneeling position advocated for lumbar surgery can give rise to air embolism, since negative pressures can occur in the vena cava with this position. Subsequently, some surgeons advocate the use of intraoperative right arterial catheters with Doppler ultrasonic transducers to monitor the possible occurrence of air embolism.[27]

INJURIES TO THE NEURAL ELEMENTS

Tears of the dura may occur during laminectomy and decompression while gaining access to the spinal canal. Packing cottonoid patties between the dura and the bony elements of the canal will prevent this mishap. Much more difficulty will be found in cases in which previous surgery has been performed with the formation of extensive scar tissue around the dura. Even with the utmost care, tears of the dura will occasionally occur. Should this injury take place, it is important to promptly repair the defect with *continuous* fine silk sutures, preferably with a noncutting needle. Failure to perform an adequate repair may result in the formation of a fistula or spinal extradural cyst.

Nerve root injuries may occur from excessive retraction, laceration, or thermal burns. Excessive retraction with metallic instruments can be avoided by gently packing the nerve roots with cotton pledgets. If this is properly performed, the nerve root can be adequately displaced medially without the necessity of repeated instrumentation, as is described in the section on the technique of disc excision. This should prevent the "battered" root syndrome that has been reported.[29]

Lacerations of the nerve root usually result from inadequate visualization and failure to recognize a flattened nerve root over an extruded disc. These injuries can be prevented with adequate visualization and careful control of bleeding. There is no particular advantage in attempting to identify a nerve root and disc herniations through a minute opening in the spinal canal. When any difficult whatsoever is encountered in recognizing the pertinent anatomic features, such as the shoulder of the nerve root and disc herniations, the laminectomy should be widened so that the nerve root can be identified with confidence proximal to the disc herniation. An excision into the annulus should never be made until the nerve root at that level is positively identified and retracted. A wide exposure, particularly laterally, will facilitate this procedure.

Thermal burns can be prevented by employing fine-tip bipolar electrocautery. However, this should be used only when the nerve root has been identified and protected. Extreme care should also be used when setting the current level, which should be checked on muscle tissue before coagulation within the spinal canal.

Complications During the Immediate Postoperative Period

These complications are not unique to spine surgery and follow the basic precepts of good surgical physiology. Pulmonary atelectasis with failure to adequately expand the lungs postoperatively is frequently seen in patients who have had endotracheal anesthesia. This occurs in the first three postoperative days and is a common cause for temperature elevations. Physical findings may be minimal and even chest radiographs may not be revealing. The best prevention and treatment are early mobilization of the patient, encouragement to cough frequently, and deep breathing. The anxious patient or patient who cannot be rapidly mobilized should routinely be placed on intermittent positive pressure breathing. Blow bottles are of some help. The authors' use of spinal anesthesia for most lumbar surgery has obviated the problem of pulmonary atelectasis to a great degree, although patient cooperation to improve ventilation is still encouraged.

INTESTINAL ILEUS

Intestinal ileus is an occasional complication of low back surgery. It will produce abdominal distention, nausea and vomiting, and respiratory distress, and auscultation will reveal the absence of bowel sounds. Treatment should include nasogastric suction with administration of intravenous fluids and electrolytes until the restoration of bowel function is indicated by peristalsis and the passage of flatus. It is our custom not to feed postlaminectomy patients for 24 hours postoperatively and to resume meals once we are confident of restitution of normal bowel function.

URINARY RETENTION

This complication is seen in the immediate postoperative course and is caused by a combination of anxiety, pain in the supine position, and nerve root irritation prior to and during surgery. The use of narcotics is also somewhat contributory to this retention. The foremost danger is the excessive use of urethral catheters, which can result in infection. Great efforts are made to manage this problem without the use of catheterization. Male patients are allowed to stand at bedside as early as the night of surgery, and female patients are allowed to use a bedside commode. If this is unsuccessful, parenteral bethanecol chloride (Urecholine) should be utilized. Only when these two measures fail is catheterization undertaken; when it is used, the intermittent variety rather than an indwelling approach has proven successful.

WOUND INFECTION

Wound infection is a complication dreaded by all surgeons. It should be suspected when pain or temperature elevation occurs during the latter part of the first postoperative week. If there is any significant suspicion of infection, the wound should be cultured either through needle aspiration or swab, and immediate Gram stain with culture and minimal inhibitory sensitivities should be obtained. If an organism is identified, treatment should be instituted immediately. In the presence of a significant infection, the patient should be returned to the operating room, and the wound should be reopened, thoroughly debrided, and irrigated. The authors prefer to leave the wound wide open and attend to daily wound care in isolation in the patient's room. If the dura is exposed, a closed irrigation system is utilized. In addition to this local care, parenteral antibiotics appropriate for the specific organism that was cultured should, of course, be administered. Areas of minor infection should be drained promptly and treated with specific antibiotics. It should be emphasized that the primary treatment of surgical infection is surgery. Antibiotics are not adequate in themselves for collections of purulent material.

In his computerized review of over 10,000 procedures, Spangfort[49] reported a postlaminectomy infection rate of approximately 2.9 per cent.

Of the more recent cases reported in his monograph, however, the infection rate had been reduced to less than 2 per cent. Occasionally, lumbar epidural abscesses will develop and characteristically will present with a progression from spinal pain to root pain to frank paresis and paralysis.[28, 41] Under this circumstance, immediate myelography, culture and sensitivity, and decompressive laminectomy would be indicated.

CAUDA EQUINA SYNDROME

This is the most dreaded complication short of death that can occur in lumbar disc surgery. The exact mechanism is uncertain, although mechanical trauma, hematoma, and vascular injury have been implicated. The artery of Adamkiewitz (arteria radicularis anteria magna) is the largest feeder of the lumbar spinal cord and has been reported entering the spinal canal between T7 and as low as the L4 level.[35] Although its predilection is for the left side between T9 and T11, injury to the vessel while retracting or cauterizing about lumbar nerves may explain this rare and unexpected complication.

Spangfort[49] reported five patients who developed a complication of cauda equina syndrome, which represented 0.2 per cent of his computerized series of patients undergoing lumbar discectomy. The severity of the syndrome is further reinforced in that only 40 per cent of these patients recovered completely.

THROMBOPHLEBITIS

Thrombophlebitis is seen with decreasing frequency since early mobilization has become routine. Its onset is heralded by a feeling of pain, tightness, and swelling in the affected extremity. Physical examination will reveal tenderness along the course of the vein and swelling of one or both extremities. A temperature elevation will frequently be seen, and a positive Homans' sign may or may not be present. Treatment with intravenous heparin, warm compresses to the leg, and elevation of the extremity is immediately instituted. The incidence of this complication is so low after spinal surgery that routine postoperative anticoagulation is not indicated unless the patient has had a prior episode of thrombophlebitis, or is obese in the extreme. Spangfort[49] reported an incidence of thrombophlebitis of only 1 per cent following laminectomy, and less than half of these patients showed any evidence of embolic phenomenon.

TECHNICAL COMPLICATIONS RESULTING IN PERSISTENT SYMPTOMS

Inadequate Nerve Root Decompression

Not infrequently, a patient continues with unrelenting sciatica postoperatively, and upon re-exploration it becomes evident that the true pathologic condition was not uncovered at the time of surgery. This complication can be prevented only if the variety of pathological entities causing nerve root compression are understood and appreciated by the surgeon. To simply look for an acute disc herniation through a small fenestration and consider this adequate treatment in all cases is to invite persistent pain. The most common conditions in which nerve root compression is not relieved are unrecognized disc lesions at another level, unrecognized lateral recess syndrome, an unappreciated migrated free fragment of disc material, foraminal encroachment, tethering of the nerve root about a pedicle, or anomalous root anatomy. These oversights can be avoided with a generous laminectomy and wide exposure whenever doubt exists as to the true nature of the pathologic state. There should be careful exploration of the nerve root from its origin at the dural sac well out into the foramen. A large, malleable cervical dilator is useful in exploring foramina. Right-angle nerve root elevators can be used with advantage to explore beneath the nerve root and dural sac and will rule out central protrusions and migrated fragments. When doubt exists as to the level of protrusion, exploration of two or three disc levels should be undertaken. An additional half hour spent in careful exploration could save the patient years of misery and disability. The importance of doing a meticulous exploration cannot be overemphasized. Parenthetically, it should be noted that no additional morbidity has been experienced with wide laminectomy.[39]

Fibrosis Around the Nerve Roots and Dura

Scar formation will occur with great regularity about the dura and nerve roots after surgical exploration. The reason for which this may cause symptoms in one patient and not in others is not understood at the present time. The scar tissue connection is a tethering as well as a constricting force about the nerve roots.

Early enthusiasm for the use of a Gelfoam membrane, advocated by LaRocca and MacNab,[43] has given way to the introduction of the concept of the free fat graft by Langenskiöld and Kiviluoto.[42] The principle of maintaining a fat-dural interface would not only inhibit perineural fibrosis and symptoms of nerve encroachment but would also allow for safer dissection if reoperation became necessary in the future. No statistical data are available yet as to the efficacy of this method; however, in the three cases personally explored by the authors where fat grafts were utilized, all were viable and little scarring was noted. More recently, Gill and others[38] suggested that a pedicle fat graft may actually be superior to the free fat graft. Careful hemostasis, as well as gentle handling of the neural tissue, will also decrease the amount of scar tissue formation.

Pseudarthrosis

Pseudarthrosis is an undesirable complication of spinal fusion. The incidence of this complication has been decreased markedly with the advent of the lateral spine fusion. In a study by DePalma and Rothman,[33] a group of 39 patients with radiographically demonstrable pseudarthrosis was studied. Of this group, only 17 per cent were symptomatic. Thus, it is the authors' recommendation that a significant trial of conservative therapy be instituted before surgical correction is undertaken. The prevention of pseudarthrosis is based on adequate surgical technique and attention to the general physiologic condition of the patient and particularly to the treatment of anemia.[48]

Disc Space Infection

Disc space infection should be considered when there is a rapid dramatic occurrence of severe back pain one to six weeks after excision of an intervertebral disc. The pain may be accompanied by recurrence of sciatica or femoral neuritis, as well as severe muscle cramping.[36] Straight leg raising or reverse straight leg raising will frequently become more limited than prior to the operation. The patient may or may not have a temperature elevation, and frequently the only laboratory abnormality would be an elevated sedimentation rate.

Serial radiographic examination will reveal loss of height of the disc space, irregular destruction of the end-plate, and ultimately, sclerotic reaction[51] (Fig. 9–22).

Diagnosis can usually be made by radiographic and clinical findings without biopsy or needle aspiration of the disc space. Treatment demands require complete immobilization, preferably in a plaster spica from the lower rib cage to above the knees. Large doses of parenteral antibiotics effective against staphylococcus organisms are utilized for a period of two to three months. However, patients who do not respond to conservative therapy within a short period of time after the institution of antibiotics should undergo debridement of the disc space either by a retroperitoneal approach or a direct posterior approach, particularly if a neurologic deficit is appreciated. Spangfort[50] estimated an incidence of approximately 2 per cent in his computerized study.

Subarachnoid Cyst

If dural tears are unrecognized or are not repaired, arachnoid cysts may form and can, on occasion, assume dramatic size. Frequently, the symptoms of an extradural pseudocyst are the same as those experienced in acute disc herniations. Occasionally, however, meningeal signs may be present, as well as headache and neck pain. Myelography will usually disclose the true nature of the patient's symptoms.[52]

Treatment of these lesions usually necessitates operation and complete excision of the cyst with closure at the dural margins either primarily or with the aid of fascial grafting. Mayfield[45] reported on 11 patients who developed this complication in a series of over 1000 operations. Most of the cases resulted from rents near the dural sleeve, and it was found that free fat plugs would successfully seal such rents.

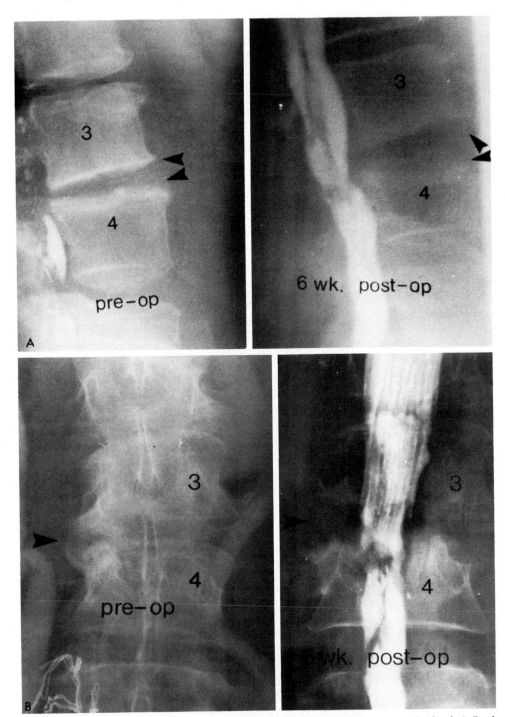

Figure 9–22. Radiographs illustrate a postoperative disc space infection at the L3-4 level. *A*, On the left preoperative lateral and on the right six weeks postoperative lateral. Note the loss of definition of the endplate and irregular destruction of the endplate and osteophytes. *B*, On the left the preoperative AP and on the right the six weeks postoperative AP revealing loss of the endplate, osteoporosis, and erosion of the osteophyte. (From Rothman, R. H., and Simeone, F. A.: The Spine, 2nd ed. Philadelphia, W. B. Saunders Co., 1982.)

Instability of a Motor Unit

Instability of a motor unit may be present preoperatively or after the excision of an intervertebral disc and associated facet joints. There is some evidence to suggest that this instability is associated with failure of relief of symptoms after disc excision.[37]

In the face of persistent back pain and sciatica after disc excision and radiographically proven instability, lateral spine fusion should be undertaken to stabilize the spine. The instability may be manifest in either a forward or reversed translation in the sagittal plane of one vertebral body or another or may be represented by wedging of the disc space with flexion and extension films. The potential for instability is not in itself an adequate justification for fusion of all spines after disc excision. The criteria for a combined procedure and spinal fusion are outlined in the discussion on indications for spinal surgery and the selection of the appropriate operative procedure.

Impingement Syndrome

After midline spinal fusion, certain patients develop symptoms at the site of contact of the fusion mass against the spinous processes of the vertebrae directly cranial to the fusion. The clinical picture is one of pain on extension of the spine with point tenderness at the area of impingement and usually can be demonstrated radiographically. Treatment of this entity requires section of the lower portion of the spinous process involved if local injection is not therapeutic.

Retained Foreign Bodies

With accurate sponge counts and the use of radiographic tagging of sponges and cotton pledgets, this complication should be rather rare. Occasionally a cotton pledget will become detached from its identifying string and if unrecognized may be retained in the wound. These foreign bodies may cause a local inflammatory reaction; for this reason, re-exploration and removal of the foreign body should be undertaken. Bone wax, as well as starch granules from the glove packaging, may sometimes cause a granulomatous reaction and persistent drainage from the wound. Therefore, bone wax should be used sparingly, if at all, and the starch on the gloves should be wiped off with a moist towel prior to surgery.

Iatrogenic Spinal Stenosis

As our temporal perspective increases, many instances are being noted of cauda equina compression secondary to overgrowth of lamina and fusion masses when midline fusion techniques have been utilized.[31] Not only will the bone graft material hypertrophy, but also, the lamina will appear to increase in thickness under the stimulus of decortication and grafting (see Fig. 9–7). The neural canal and foramina may be encroached, presenting a classic spinal stenotic syndrome. The clinical syndrome is usually quite apparent, but computerized axial tomography may provide a diagnostic clue as to this entity. Treatment in either case would require satisfactory decompression of the neural elements.

Pelvic Instability

The creation of pelvic instability after removing iliac bone for grafting and fatigue fractures at the site of the bone removed are rare complications of spinal fusion but should be considered in patients with persistent back pain after fusion.[32] Fatigue fractures will heal spontaneously. Symptomatic pelvic instability may require a sacroiliac fusion.

THE SURGICAL TREATMENT OF SPONDYLOLISTHESIS IN ADULTS

The clinical picture of spondylolisthesis evolves gradually as one studies the transition from late adolescence to early adulthood.

Spondylolisthesis merits discussion in a chapter dealing with lumbar disc disease, since Type III[76] (degenerative spondylolisthesis) (Table 9–9) is secondary to degenerative changes in the intervertebral disc and the facet joint with subsequent motion segment instability.[55, 59, 62, 66] Furthermore, any of the classified forms of spondylolisthesis not only can give rise to low back pain syndromes but also can contribute to a radicular syndrome and the intermittent neurogenic claudication syndrome, which were discussed previously.[62]

TABLE 9–9. Types of Spondylolisthesis

I—Dysplastic—In this type of congenital abnormality, the upper sacrum or arch of L5 permits the olisthesis to occur.

II—Isthmic—The lesion is in the pars interarticularis. Three types can be recognized.
    a. Lytic—fatigue fracture of the pars
    b. Elongated but intact pars
    c. Acute fracture

III—Degenerative—resulting from long-standing intersegmental instability.

IV—Traumatic—resulting from fractures in other areas of the bony hook and the pars.

V—Pathologic—There is generalized or localized bone disease.

Type I and Type II

It is important to differentiate the clinical syndrome and pathologic condition in the skeletally immature spine from that found in the adult. In the former, the growth potential merits different management.[58, 77]

Upon reaching maturity, the fear of further anterior migration of Type I and Type II spondylolisthesis is no longer present and is only a minor consideration in terms of surgical treatment.

There is, however, significant evidence that individuals with a pars defect will have a 25 per cent greater likelihood of back disability than an individual without the defect.[60, 72, 78] MacNab,[62] after studying 1000 patients with back pain, concluded that spondylolisthesis is most likely the cause of pain in patients under 26 years of age but rarely the sole cause of complaints after the age of 40. The various pain syndromes that can occur are most likely caused by disc degeneration, presumably resulting from abnormal movement between the involved motion segments.[67]

The mechanical stresses, particularly torsional stresses, that are most detrimental to the disc are exerted upon the annulus, with resultant early breakdown. Interestingly enough, extrusion of nuclear material at this level is very uncommon. In the authors' experience with the operative treatment of spondylolisthesis, extrusions have been noted above the level of the spondylolisthesis but only rarely at the same level. Scoville and others,[71] however, described 11 to 15 patients with a herniation occurring at the same level as the spondylolisthesis.

After emphasizing the usual forms of nonoperative therapy, such as limitation of stressful activities, lumbosacral corseting, and spinal and abdominal exercises, certain individuals will remain incapacitated by low back pain and leg pain secondary to spondylolisthesis. These individuals should be considered as candidates for surgery.[64] Progressive deformity and neurologic deficit are subsidiary considerations in terms of management decisions.

It is unrealistic to recommend any one surgical procedure for the entire spectrum of clinical disorders associated with spondylolisthesis. Great confusion has existed in the literature. Advocates can be found for simple nerve root decompression by resection of the loose neural arch for Type I (many can have associated pars defects) and Type II slips with or without fusion. When selecting the optimal type of surgical treatment, the physician must consider the age of the patient, his functional demands, the clinical pain pattern, evidence of dynamic instability, and the anatomic configuration of the spine (type of olisthesis) in regard to degree of slip and size of the transverse processes. The decision to fuse may also depend on the degree of iatrogenic instability created intraoperatively in order to achieve satisfactory neural decompression.

Despite the frequent occurrence of this disorder and the high number of surgical procedures performed on an annual basis, there are no randomized prospective studies in the literature of the surgical treatment of spondylolisthesis. In the absence of this essential information, the surgeon must be guided by personal experience and skill as well as by the limited amount of information that is available from the retrospective studies conducted in the literature.

A plan of approach to this problem in adults is outlined below; the authors have found it to be generally satisfactory, and it has been supported by the work of others interested in this problem.

BACK PAIN ONLY

The existence of spondylolisthesis and of spondylolysis has been correlated with lumbosacral complaints.[65, 74] The source of back pain is not certain, but a recent anatomic investigation of 485 skeletons by Eisenstein[54] found, without exception, abnormally enlarged superior facets of the affected spondylytic vertebra in the 3.5 per cent of involved specimens, implicating facet overload as a pain pathway in Type II olisthesis. Most patients with spondylolisthesis have back pain and lumbar insufficiency as primary symptoms. Approximately one third will have sciatica in addition, a ratio constant in both children and adults.[61] A successful spinal fusion will usually alleviate symptoms in individuals who have only back pain.[57, 70, 73] The relief of pain with solid fusion is most effectively achieved by the technique of posterolateral fusion, since it provides for a large graft bed with inclusion of the facet joints and incidental obliteration of the medial branch of the posterior rami as it courses over the intersection of the transverse process and the superior facet of the involved vertebra.[69] The extent of the fusion will depend on both the degree of slip and the size of the fifth transverse process. When the degree of slip is minor and the fifth transverse process is large, the fusion need extend only from L5 to the sacrum.[79] If the degree of slip is large and the transverse process is small, the fusion should be carried from the sacrum to the fourth transverse process. When there is any doubt as to the adequacy of the transverse process, the surgeon should not hesitate to extend the fusion to L4 in order to obtain a more adequate bed.

BACK PAIN AND LEG PAIN

Those skeletally mature individuals with both back and leg pain require both central and foraminal decompression by excision of the loose neural arch and the fibrocartilaginous mass at the defect site and stabilization of the spine by fusion for optimal relief of symptoms. This appears to combine the excellent relief of sciatica produced by decompression, as advocated by Gill and colleagues, with the stability and relief of back pain offered by spinal fusion.[56]

Osterman and others[68] provided long-term follow-up study on patients who underwent the Gill procedure without stabilization and found an unsatisfactory result in 19 of 75 patients between the ages of 30 and 59. They attributed the rise from 17 per cent unsatisfactory results after one year to 25 per cent after five years to disc degeneration that they noted roentgenographically at the level of the decompression.

The combined procedure, therefore, is the operation used most commonly by the authors for symptomatic spondylolisthesis in the physiologically young or functionally active adult. It has yielded excellent results in our hands as well as in others: Rombold[70] reported 93 per cent satisfactory long-term result with this approach. As previously stated, the extent of the fusion should be determined by the size and accessibility of the fifth transverse process.

PATIENTS OVER AGE 60 WITH PREDOMINANT LEG PAIN

In older patients in whom leg pain is a predominant symptom, simple resection of the loose posterior elements and nerve root compression as advocated by Gill appears to be a satisfactory approach. At times, resection of the caudal portion of the ventral part of the pedicle may also be necessary to adequately decompress the spinal nerve.[75] The enthusiastic reports by Gill for the treatment of spondylolisthesis have not been uniformly supported. Amuso and coauthors[53] noted only 65 per cent satisfactory results using the same criteria for grading as Gill; however, older individuals with limited demands on the spine and greater intrinsic stability at the level of the spondylolisthesis will usually obtain satisfactory relief of pain. Further progression of the slip after resection of the posterior elements, a valid fear in children, does not appear to be a problem in adults.[53, 56] Indeed, although Osterman[68] and Vestad and Naes[75] reported progression of olisthesis in many skeletally mature patients (the increased slip actually decreasing in absolute terms with increasing age) subjected to decompression only, neither reported any correlation between the final results and the degree of postoperative slip.

NONUNION OF SPINAL FUSION

It is recommended that those individuals who have a pseudarthrosis after a midline spinal fusion and whose symptoms justify the need for further surgery have a lateral spine fusion. In patients who have had a lateral spine fusion that has failed, the anterior approach to the spine is utilized (see Anterior Interbody Fusion). If the primary approach to the spondylolisthesis has been the anterior approach and nonunion has resulted, a posterolateral spine fusion is undertaken.

Type III Degenerative Spondylolisthesis

Degenerative spondylolisthesis (and retro-olisthesis) represents a true migration of one vertebral body on another in the sagittal plane but does not represent the true defect in the posterior neural arch. Rather, malalignment of the vertebrae is associated with and caused by disc degeneration and instability of both the disc itself and the facet joints subjected to static and dynamic forces acting in the lumbar spine. For discussion of this relationship, the reader is referred to the section dealing with intermittent claudication in Chapter 1. The surgical treatment of the disorder is considered together with disc degeneration and spinal stenosis.

Type IV and Type V spondylolisthesis are unusual types of olisthesis that merit individualized management beyond the scope of this chapter. The principles that guide treatment, however, which are similar to those applicable to the other forms of spondylolisthesis, rest on diagnosis, relief of pain (both osseous and neural in origin), and stabilization.

REFERENCES

INDICATIONS FOR SURGERY

1. Caldwell, A. B., and Chase, C.: Diagnosis and treatment of personality factors in chronic low back pain. Clin. Orthop., *129*:141, 1977.
2. Hanvick, L. J.: MMPI profiles in patients with low back pain. J. Consult. Psychol., *15*:350, 1951.
3. Hirsch, C.: Efficiency of surgery in low back disorders. J. Bone Joint Surg., *47A*:991, 1965.
4. Maruta, T., Swanson, D. V., and Swenson, W. M.: Low back pain patients in a psychiatric population. Mayo Clin. Proc., *51*:57, 1976.
5. Maury, M., Francois, N., and Skoda, A.: About the neurological sequelae of herniated intervertebral disc. Paraplegia, *11*:221, 1973.
6. Mooney, V., Cairns, D., and Robertson, J.: A system for evaluating and treating chronic back disability. West. J. Med., *5*:370, 1976.
7. Ransford, A. O., Cairns, D., and Mooney, V.: The pain drawing as an aid to the psychologic evaluation of patients with low back pain. Spine, *2*:127, 1976.
8. Weber, H.: Lumbar disc herniation: A prospective study of prognostic factors including a controlled trial. J. Oslo City Hosp., *28*:33,89, 1978.
9. Wiltse, L. L., and Rocchio, P. D.: Pre-operative psychological tests as predictors of success of chemonucleolysis treatment of the low back syndrome. J. Bone Joint Surg., *57A*:478, 1975.
10. Wolkind, S. N.: Psychiatric aspects of low back pain. Psychotherapy, *3*:75, 1974.

INDICATIONS FOR FUSION

11. Semmes, E.: Ruptures of the Lumbar Intervertebral Disc. Springfield, Charles C Thomas Co., 1964.
12. Young, H., and Love, J.: End results of removal of protruded lumbar intervertebral discs with and without fusion. AAOS Instructional Course Lecture, *16*:213, 1959.

SURGICAL TECHNIQUES

13. DiStefano, V. J., et al.: Intraoperative analysis of the effects of position body habitus on surgery of the low back. Clin. Orthop., *99*:51, 1974.

LUMBAR DECOMPRESSIVE LAMINECTOMY AND FORAMINOTOMY

14. McNab, I.: The laminectomy membrane. J. Bone Joint Surg., *56B*:545, 1974.
15. Langenskiöld, A., and Kiviluoto, O.: Prevention of epidural scar formation after operation on the lumbar spine by means of a free fat transplant. Clin. Orthop., *115*:92, 1976.
16. Gill, G. C., et al.: Pedicle fat graft for the prevention of scar formation after laminectomy. Proceedings of the 5th Annual Meeting of the International Society for the Study of the Lumbar Spine. San Francisco, 1978.
17. Jacobs, R., McClain, O., and Neff, J.: Control of post-laminectomy scar formation: An experimental and clinical evaluation. Spine *5*:223, 1980.

LATERAL SPINE FUSION

18. DePalma, A., and Rothman, R.: The Intervertebral Disc. Philadelphia, W. B. Saunders Co., 1970.

19. Truchly, G., et al.: Posterolateral fusion of the lumbosacral spine. J. Bone Joint Surg., *44A*:505, 1962.
20. Watkins, M. B.: Lumbosacral fusion results with early ambulation. Surg. Gynecol. Obstet., *102*:604, 1956.

ANTERIOR INTERBODY FUSION

21. Harmon, P. H., and Abel, M.: Correlation of multiple objective diagnostic methods in lower lumbar disc disease. Clin. Orthop., *28*:132, 1963.
22. Goldner, J. L., et al.: Anterior disc excision and interbody spine fusion for chronic low back pain. Orthop. Clin. North Am., *2*:543, 1971.

RESULTS OF OPERATIVE TREATMENT OF LUMBAR DISC DISEASE

23. DePalma, A., and Rothman, R.: Surgery of the lumbar spine. Clin. Orthop., *63*:162, 1969.
24. Knutsson, B.: Aspects of the neurogenic electromyographic records of voluntary contraction in cases of nerve root compression. Electromyography, *2*:238, 1962.
25. Hirsch, C.: Efficiency of surgery in low back disorders. J. Bone Joint Surg., *47A*:991, 1965.
26. DePalma, A., and Rothman, R.: The nature of pseudarthrosis. Clin. Orthop., *59*:113, 1968.

COMPLICATIONS

27. Albin, M. S.: Venous air embolism and lumbar disk surgery. Letter to the Editor. JAMA, *240*:1713, 1978.
28. Baker, A. S., Ojemann, R. G., Schwartz, M. N., and Richardson, E. P.: Spinal epidural abscess. N. Engl. J. Med., *293*:463, 1975.
29. Bertrand, G.: The "battered" root problem. Orthop. Clin. North Am., *6*:305, 1975.
30. Birkeland, I. W., and Taylor, T. K. F.: Major vascular injuries in lumbar disc surgery. J. Bone Joint Surg., *51B*:4, 1969.
31. Brodsky, A. E.: Post-laminectomy and post-fusion stenosis of the lumbar spine. Clin. Orthop., *115*:130, 1976.
32. Coventry, M. B., and Tapper, E.: Pelvic instability. J. Bone Joint Surg., *54A*:83, 1972.
33. DePalma, A., and Rothman, R.: The nature of pseudarthrosis. Clin. Orthop., *59*:113, 1968.
34. Desausseure, R. L.: Vascular injuries coincident to disc surgery. J. Neurosurg., *16*:222, 1959.
35. Dommise, G. F.: The blood supply of the spinal cord. J. Bone Joint Surg., *56B*:225, 1974.
36. El-Gindi, S., Aref, S., Salama, M., and Andrew, J.: Infection of intervertebral discs after operation. J. Bone Joint Surg., *58*:114, 1976.
37. Froning, E. C., and Frohman, B.: Motion of the lumbosacral spine after laminectomy and spine fusion. J. Bone Joint Surg., *50A*:897, 1968.
38. Gill, G. C., Sakovich, L., and Thompson, E.: Pedicle fat graft for the prevention of scar formation after laminectomy: An experimental study in dogs. Proceedings of the 5th Annual Meeting of the International Society for the Study of the Lumbar Spine. San Francisco, 1978.
39. Jackson, R. K.: The long-term effects of wide laminectomy for lumbar disc excision. J. Bone Joint Surg., *53B*:609, 1971.
40. Jarstfer, B. S., and Rich, N. M.: The challenge of arteriovenous fistula formation following disk surgery: A collective review. J. Trauma, *16*:726, 1976.
41. Keon-Cohen, B. T.: Epidural abscess simulating disc herniation. J. Bone Joint Surg., *50B*:128, 1968.
42. Langenskiöld, A., and Kiviluoto, O.: Prevention of epidural scar formation after operations on the lumbar spine by means of free fat transplants. Clin. Orthop., *115*:92, 1976.
43. LaRocca, H., and MacNab, I.: The laminectomy membrane. J. Bone Joint Surg., *56B*:545, 1974.
44. Lindblom, K.: Intervertebral disc degeneration as a pressure atrophy. J. Bone Joint Surg., *39A*:933, 1957.
45. Mayfield, F. H.: Complications of laminectomy. Clin. Neurosurg., *23*:435, 1976.
46. Montorsi, W., and Chiringhelli, C.: Genesis, diagnosis and treatment of vascular complications after intervertebral disc surgery. Int. Surg., *58*:233, 1973.

47. Moore, C. A., and Cohen, A.: Combined arterial venous and urethral injuries complicating disc surgery. Am. J. Surg., *115*:574, 1968.
48. Rothman, R., et al.: The effect of iron deficiency anemia on fracture healing. Clin. Orthop., 77:276, 1971.
49. Spangfort, E. V.: The lumbar disc herniation — A computerized analysis of 2504 Operations. Acta. Orthop. Scand. Suppl., *142*:52, 1972.
50. Spangfort, E. V.: Postoperative discitis. Nord. Med., *71*:162, 1964.
51. Thibodeau, A. A.: Closed space infection following removal of lumbar intervertebral disc. J. Bone Joint Surg., *50A*:400, 1968.
52. Borgesen, S. E., and Vang, P. S.: Extradural pseudocysts. A cause of pain after lumbar disc operation. Acta Orthop. Scand., *44*:12, 1973.

SPONDYLOLISTHESIS

53. Amuso, S. et al.: The surgical treatment of spondylolisthesis by posterior element resection. J. Bone Joint Surg., *52A*:529, 1970.
54. Eisenstein, S.: The morphology and pathological anatomy of the lumbar spine in South African Negroes and Caucasoids with specific reference to spinal stenosis. J. Bone Joint Surg., *59B*:173, 1977.
55. Fitzgerald, J. A. W., and Newman, P. H.: Degenerative spondylolisthesis. J. Bone Joint Surg., *58B*:184, 1976.
56. Gill, G., Manning, J. G., and White, H. L.: Surgical treatment of spondylolisthesis without spine fusion. J. Bone Joint Surg., *37A*:493, 1955.
57. Henderson, E. D.: Results of the surgical treatment of spondylolisthesis. J. Bone Joint Surg., *48A*:619, 1966.
58. Hensinger, R. N., Lang, J. R., and MacEwen, G. D.: Surgical management of spondylolisthesis in children and adolescents. Spine *1*:207, 1976.
59. Junghanns, H.: Spondyolisthesen ohne Spalt im Zwischengelenstuck. Archiv fur Orthopadische and Unfall-Chirurgie, *29*:118, 1930–31.
60. Kettelkamp, D., and Wright, D.: Spondylolisthesis in the Alaskan Eskimo. Paper presented at the Meeting of the Western Orthopedic Association. Portland, Oregon, October 6, 1970.
61. Laurent, L., and Einola, S.: Spondylolisthesis in children and adolescents. Acta. Orthop. Scand., *31*:45, 1961.
62. MacNab, I.: Spondylolisthesis with an intact neural arch — The so-called pseudospondylolisthesis. J. Bone Joint Surg., *32B*:325, 1950.
63. MacNab, I.: Backache. Baltimore, Williams & Wilkins Co., 1977.
64. Magora, A.: Conservative treatment in spondylolisthesis. Clin. Orthop., *117*:74, 1976.
65. Nachemson, A.: The lumbar spine. An orthopaedic challenge. Spine, *1*:59, 1976.
66. Newman, P. H., and Stone, K. H.: The etiology of spondylolisthesis. J. Bone Joint Surg., *45B*:39, 1963.
67. Olsson, T. H., Selvik, G., and Willner, S.: Vertebral motion in spondylolisthesis. Acta. Radiol. [Diagn], 17(6):861, 1976.
68. Osterman, K., Lindholm, M. D., and Laurent, L. E.: Late results of removal of the loose posterior element (Gill's operation) in the treatment of the lytic lumbar spondylolisthesis. Clin. Orthop. *117*:121, 1976.
69. Penderson, H. E., Blunk, L. F. J., and Gardner, E.: Anatomy of lumbosacral posterior rami and meningeal branches of spinal nerves. J. Bone Joint Surg., *38A*:377, 1956.
70. Rombold, C.: Treatment of spondylolisthesis by posterolateral fusion. J. Bone Joint Surg., *48A*:1282, 1966.
71. Scoville, W. B., and Corkell, G.: Lumbar spondylolisthesis with ruptured disc. J. Neurosurg., *40*:529, 1974.
72. Splitoff, C.: Roentgenographic comparison of patients with and without backache. J.A.M.A., *152*:1610, 1953.
73. Stauffer, R., and Coventry, M.: Posterolateral lumbar spine fusion. J. Bone Joint Surg., *54A*:1195, 1972.
74. Jorgensen, W. R., and Dotter, W. E.: Comparative roentgenographic study of the asymptomatic and symptomatic lumbar spine. J. Bone Joint Surg., *58A*:850, 1976.
75. Vestad, E., and Naes, B.: Spondylolisthesis. Acta. Orthop. Scand., *48*:472, 1977.
76. Wiltse, L. L., and Newman, P. H., and MacNab, I.: Classification of spondylolysis and spondylolisthesis. Clin. Orthop., *117*:23, 1976.
77. Wiltse, L. L., and Jacobson, D. W.: Treatment of spondylolisthesis and spondylolysis in children. Clin. Orthop., *117*:92, 1976.
78. Wiltse, L. L.: The effect of common anomalies of the lumbar spine upon disc degeneration and low back pain. Orthop. Clin. North Am., 2:569, 1971.
79. Wiltse, L. L., and Hutchison, R.: Surgical treatment of spondylolisthesis. Clin. Orthop., *35*:116, 1964.

APPENDIX OF SPINAL TERMS

The American Academy of Orthopedic Surgeons has completed a glossary on spinal terminology. It is hoped that this will lead to the standardization of spinal nomenclature. Only the sections that apply to the lumbar spine have been included in this text. We would like to thank the American Academy of Orthopedic Surgeons for granting us permission to include these terms.

ANATOMIC TERMS

PLATE 1. LATERAL VIEW OF THE FIRST AND FOURTH THORACIC VERTEBRAE AND AXIAL VIEW OF TYPICAL LUMBAR VERTEBRA.

1. Circular fovea for first rib.
2. Costal fovea of transverse process.
3. Pedicle.
4. Inferior costal fovea.
5. Superior articular facet on superior articular process.
6. Spine.
7. Vertebral body.
8. Superior costal fovea.
9. Mamillary process.
10. Accessory process.
11. Transverse process.
12. Annular epiphysis.
13. Vertebral body.
14. Lateral recess of vertebral foramen.
15. Vertebral arch. Pars interarticularis (not shown) is the part of the neural arch between the superior and inferior articular processes.

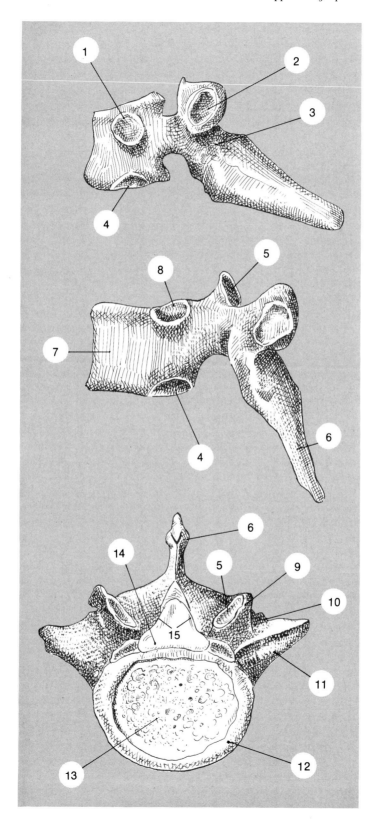

PLATE 2. OBLIQUE OF THORACIC VERTEBRAE.

1. Superior vertebral notch.
2. Transverse process.
3. Superior articular facet.
4. Superior costal fovea.
5. Facet joint (zygoapophyseal joint).
6. Spinous process.
7. Costal fovea of transverse process.
8. Inferior articular process.
9. Inferior vertebral notch.
10. Inferior costal fovea.
11. Vertebral foramen.
12. Vertebral canal.
13. Intervertebral foramen.

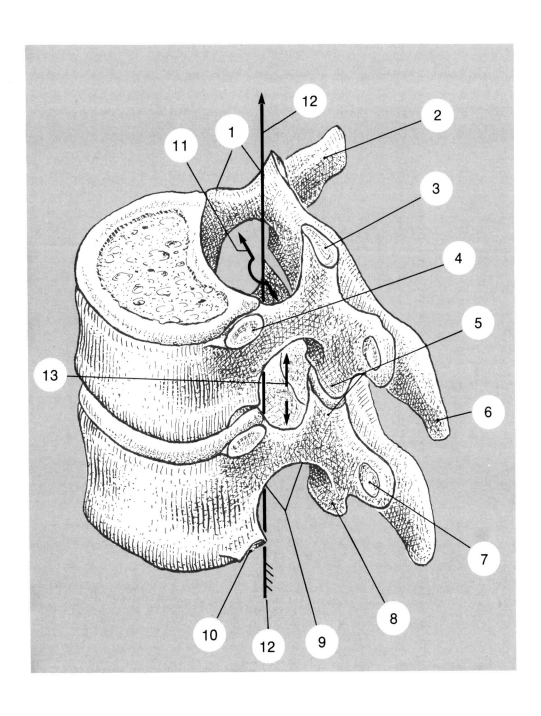

PLATE 3. DORSAL AND VENTRAL COMPOSITE OF SACRUM AND LIGAMENTS OF THE SACROCOCCYGEAL JOINT.

1. Superior articular facet on superior articular process.
2. Auricular surface.
2.5 Intermediate sacral crest.
3. Lateral sacral crest.
4. Median sacral crest.
5. Fourth dorsal sacral foramina.
6. Sacral horns.
7. Sacral hiatus.
8. Transverse line.
9. Pelvic sacral foramina.
10. Pelvic surface.
11. Sacral promontory.
12. Lateral part.
13. Base of sacrum.
14. Sacral canal.
15. Sacrococcygeal joint.
16. Coccygeal horns.
17. Deep dorsal sacrococcygeal ligament.
18. Superficial dorsal sacrococcygeal ligament.
19. Lateral sacrococcygeal ligament.

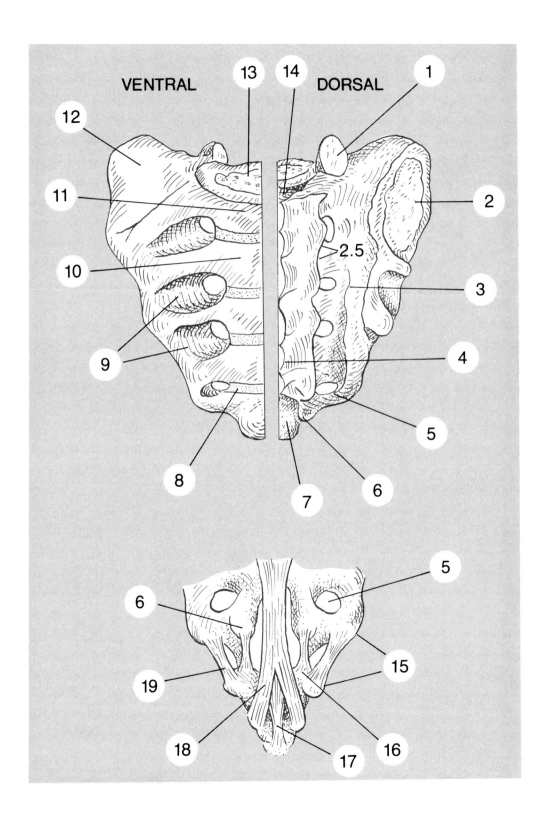

PLATE 4. ARTERIAL SUPPLY TO CORD AND ROOTS.

1. Dorsolateral longitudinal artery.
2. Proximal radicular artery (of dorsal root).
3. Dorsal medullary artery.
4. Dorsal root of spinal nerve.
5. Distal radicular artery (of dorsal root).
6. Sinuvertebral nerve.
7. Dorsal ramus of spinal nerve.
8. Segmental artery.
9. Posterior central artery.
10. Dorsal root ganglion.
11. Anterior laminar artery.
12. Ventral ramus of spinal nerve.
13. White and gray rami to sympathetic ganglia.
14. Ventral root of spinal nerve.
15. Proximal radicular artery of ventral root.
16. Periradicular sheath of dura.
17. Dorsal meningeal branch of spinal artery.
18. Dura.
19. Ventral meningeal plexus.
20. Great ventral medullary artery.
21. Ventral longitudinal spinal artery.
22. Vasa corona of spinal cord.
23. Spinal nerves.
24. Ventral medullary artery.

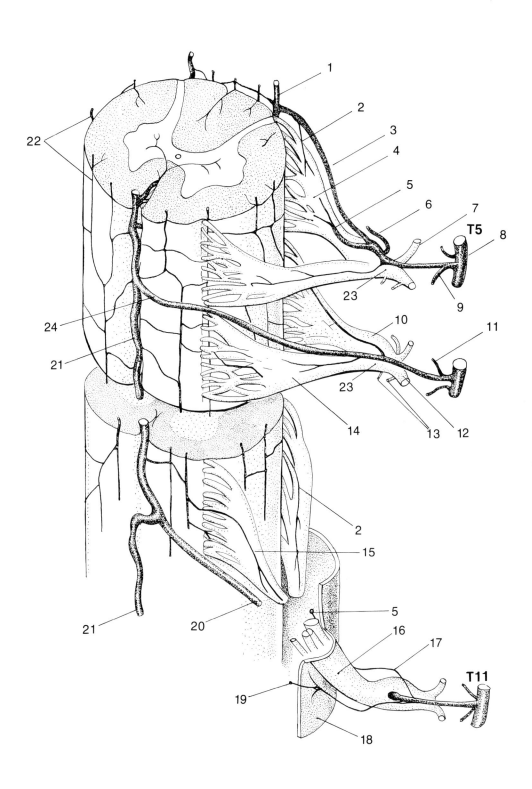

PLATE 5. VERTEBRAL VEINS.

1. Dorsal external vertebral venous plexus.
2. Dorsal internal vertebral venous plexus.
3. Intervertebral vein.
4. Basivertebral vein.
5. Ventral external vertebral venous plexus.
6. Segmental vein.
7. Lateral (lumbar or intercostal) branch.
8. Dorsal branch of segmental vein.
9. Ventral internal vertebral venous plexus.
10. Venous ring of internal venous plexuses.

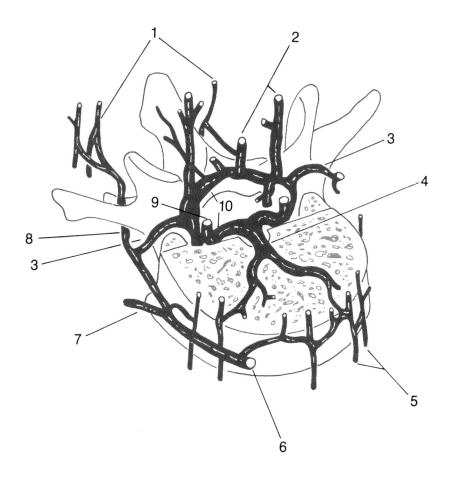

PLATE 6. SCHEMA OF HEMISECTION OF VERTEBRAL COLUMN ILLUSTRATING RELATIONS OF MENINGES TO COLUMN, CORD, AND SPINAL NERVES.

1. Epidural space.
2. Dura.
3. Subdural space.
4. Arachnoid.
5. Subarachnoid space.
6. Pia forming dentate ligament. (The sides of dentate ligaments form the two denticulate ligaments that extend almost the entire length of the cord on each side.)
7. The true spinal nerve.*
8. Intravaginal parts of the dorsal and ventral spinal roots.
9. Interradicular foramen.
10. Dorsal primary ramus of spinal nerve.
11. Ventral primary ramus of spinal nerve.
12. Rami communicantes.

---

*A segment of the nerve proximal to the ganglion yet outside the main dural sac is the preganglionic spinal nerve whereas that beyond the ganglion is called the postganglionic spinal nerve, the two segments making up the true spinal nerve.

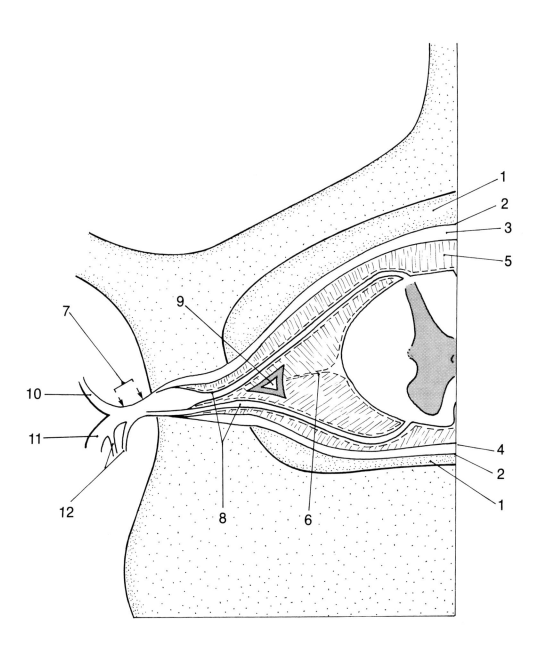

PLATE 7. SCHEMA OF DISTRIBUTION OF POSTERIOR CENTRAL BRANCHES OF SPINAL BRANCHES OF THE SEGMENTAL ARTERIES AND THE DISTRIBUTION OF THE SINUVERTEBRAL NERVES TO THE DISCS AND VERTEBRAL BODIES.

1. Dorsal root ganglion (retracted).
2. Rami communicantes.
3. Sinuvertebral nerve.
4. Intravaginal parts of dorsal and ventral spinal nerve roots.
5. Spinal nerve.
6. Dorsal primary ramus of spinal nerve.
7. Ventral primary ramus of spinal nerve.
8. Foramen of the basivertebral vein.
9. Posterior longitudinal plexus of posterior central arteries.
10. Spinal branch of segmental artery.
11. Extent of intervertebral foramen.
12. Lateral recess of vertebral (spinal) canal.
13. Posterior longitudinal ligament.

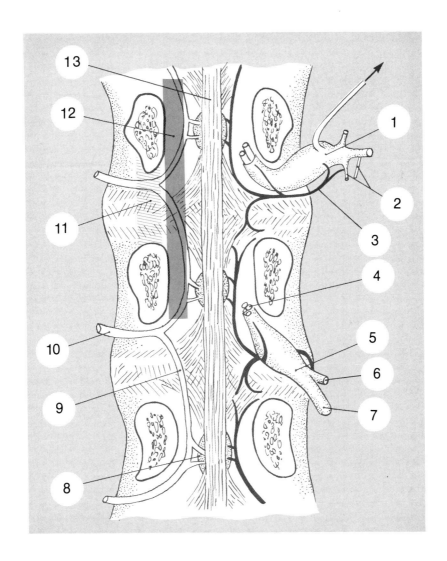

PLATE 8. SCHEMA OF SAGITTAL SECTION OF SPINE SHOWING CONTENTS OF INTERVERTEBRAL FORAMEN IN RELATION TO DISC AND MOTOR SEGMENT UNIT.

1. Articular capsule of facet joint.
2. Intervertebral vein(s).
3. Ligamentum flavum.
4. Dorsal root ganglion and ventral spinal root within vaginal extension of dura accompanied by radicular vein.
5. Sinuvertebral nerve.
6. Spinal branch of segmental artery.
7. Perforated chondral plate of vertebral body that permits nutrient perfusions to reach tissues of the disc.
8. Nucleus pulposus.
9. Ring apophysis of vertebral body.
10. Annulus.

A. Motor segment unit as originally proposed by Junghanns.

B-B. Motor segment (motion segment) unit as proposed by Parke to include all components of original somite.

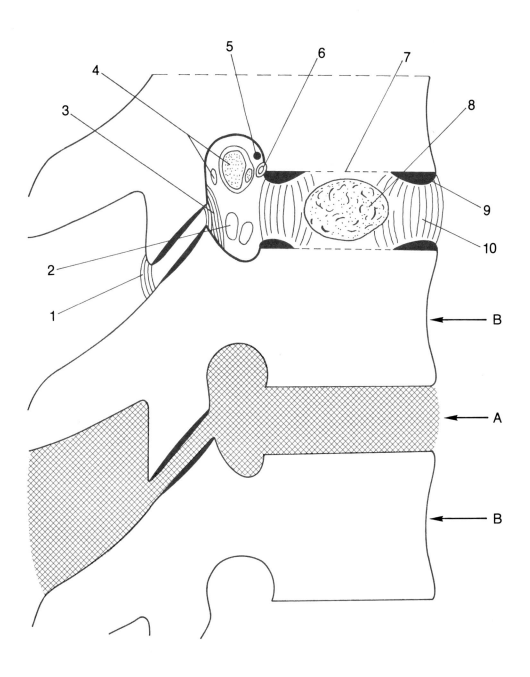

PATHOLOGIC TERMS

Ankylosing Spinal Hyperostosis (Forestier's Disease): An arthritic disorder in which bridging osteophytes located anteriorly and laterally on the vertebral body bind two or more vertebrae together.

Ankylosing Spondylitis (Marie-Strümpell Disease): An inflammatory disease of the spine that leads to bony ankylosis of the vertebral articulations.

Arachnoiditis: Arachnoidal inflammatory disease leading to fibrosis that binds the roots of the cauda equina.

Cervical Spondylosis: Degenerative disease of both the disc and the zygapophyseal joints, occurring in the cervical spine.

Degenerative Disc Disease: That disorder in which disc degeneration produces clinical symptoms and signs.

Degenerative Joint Disease of the Zygapophyseal Joint (Facet Arthrosis): Degenerative changes in the zygapophyseal joints characterized by cartilage thinning and osteophyte formation.

Diastematomyelia: An embryologic spinal defect in which the spinal cord or the cauda equina is divided by a cartilaginous or bony mass located in the midsagittal region of the spinal canal.

Disc Degeneration: The loss of the structural and functional integrity of the disc.

Discitis: An inflammatory disorder of the intervertebral disc.

Dysraphism: Any failure of closure of the primary neural tube.

Epineural Fibrosis (Root Sleeve Fibrosis): Scar tissue surrounding a spinal nerve root in the spinal canal or neural foramen.

Facet Tropism: Asymmetric orientation of the facets of the right and left zygapophyseal joints of a vertebral articulation.

Herniated Nucleus Pulposus (Intervertebral Disc Rupture): Displacement of nuclear material and other disc components beyond the normal confines of the annulus. Four degrees of displacement are recognized:
Intraspongy nuclear herniation

Protrusion: The displaced material causes a discrete bulge in the annulus, but no material escapes through the annular fibers.

Extrusion: The displaced material presents in the spinal canal through disrupted fibers of the annulus but remains connected to material persisting within the disc.

Sequestration: Nuclear material escapes into the spinal canal as a free fragment(s) that may migrate to other locations.

Interspinous Pseudarthrosis: The development of a false joint between two spinous processes.

Intraneural Fibrosis: Scar tissue within the substance of a spinal nerve.

Juvenile Osteochondrosis (Juvenile Epiphysitis, Scheuermann's Disease): Disorder of the secondary vertebral ring apophyses that may produce wedging or other changes of the vertebral bodies.

Limbus Annulare: A mass of bone situated at the anterosuperior margin of a vertebra that arises from failure of fusion of the primary and secondary ossification centers.

Myelitis: Inflammatory disease of the spinal cord producing symptoms and signs of cord dysfunction.

Myelopathy: Noninflammatory disease of the spinal cord producing symptoms and signs of cord dysfunction.

Osteopenia: Any state in which bone mass is reduced below normal.

Osteomalacia: Reduction in the physical strength of bone resulting from decreased mineralization of osteoid.

Osteoporosis: Diminution in both the mineral and matrix components of bone.

Pseudarthrosis: A defect in bone secondary to failure of union in either a bone or bone graft.

Radiculitis: Inflammation of a spinal nerve in the spinal canal or neural canal.

Radiculopathy: Noninflammatory abnormality of a spinal nerve in the spinal canal or neural foramen resulting in neurologic deficit.

Retrolisthesis: Posterior displacement of a vertebra on the one below.

Segmental Instability: An abnormal response to applied loads characterized by motion in the motor segment beyond normal constraints.

Spinal Stenosis: Reduction in the size of the spinal canal or regions thereof to a pathologic degree. The classifications are:
Congenital Stenosis: Malformation present at birth.

Developmental Stenosis: Malformation of genetic origin.

Acquired Stenosis: Malformation developed after birth. It is a lateral stenosis of the nerve canal (lateral recess entrapment).

Spondylitis: An inflammatory disease of the spine.

Spondylolisthesis: Anterior displacement of a vertebra on the adjacent vertebra below, which occurs in one of five types:

Dysplastic: The orientation of the facets of the zygapophyseal joint is sufficiently horizontal to permit slipping, or the superior facet of the lower vertebra is hypoplastic, thus attaining displacement of the upper vertebrae.

Isthmic: Fibrous defects are present in the pars interarticularis that permit forward displacement of the upper vertebrae and separation of the anterior aspects of that vertebra from its neural arch.

Degenerative: Anterior displacement of a vertebra arising from erosive degenerative changes in the zygapophyseal joints.

Traumatic: Anterior displacement of a vertebra caused by traumatic injury to its restraining structures.

Pathologic: Anterior displacement of a vertebra because of elongation of the pedicles from a disease process in the bone.

Spondylolysis: A defect in the pars interarticularis.

Spondylosis: Degenerative disease of both the disc and the zygapophyseal joints.

Traction Spur: A bony excrescence appearing on the anterolateral surface of the vertebral body near but not at the·body margin that arises as a result of disc degeneration.

Transitional Vertebra: A vertebra whose structure features some of the characteristics of both of two adjacent spinal regions.

Vacuum Phenomenon: The presence of an air shadow within an intervertebral disc on roentgenogram.

Vertebral Osteomyelitis: Infection in the bony structures of the spine.

CLINICAL TERMS

CLINICAL SIGNS AND TESTS:

Straight leg raising test: With the patient lying supine with both lower limbs extended and relaxed, the extremity is raised, normally 70 to 90 degrees without discomfort. The test is positive when this maneuver elicits ipsilateral sciatic limb pain.

Lasègue's Test: This is the second maneuver described by Forst. After performing the straight leg raising test, the limb is flexed at the hip and knee while the foot is allowed to slide toward the buttocks. In the presence of radiculopathy, sciatic pain is produced by the straight leg raising and is relieved when Lasègue's test is performed. Lasègue's test is painless in sciatica and painful in hip disease.

Kernig's Sign: This sign is elicited with the patient lying supine. The examiner first flexes the hip and then extends the knee. Normally, knee extension is possible to 135 degrees. The test is positive when knee extension is limited and painful. It indicates the presence of meningeal irritation but is also positive in lumbar disc protrusion on the side of sciatic pain.

Patrick's "F-AB-ER-E" Sign: The patient lies supine and the heel of the lower limb being tested is passively placed on the opposite knee as high above the patella as possible. The knee on the side being tested is then pressed laterally and downward by the examiner. The test is considered positive if motion is involuntarily restricted and hip pain is produced. The test is positive in hip joint disease and negative in sciatica. F-ab-er-e stands for flexion (f), abduction (ab), external rotation (er), and extension (e).

Foot-Dorsiflexion Test: This test is a refinement of the straight leg raising test. Once gentle elevation of an affected limb produces sciatic pain, slow or brisk dorsiflexion of the foot intensifies it.

Bow-String Sign (Cram Test):   This was described by Gower as follows: "Let the patient sit on a chair with the knee at a little more than right angle and the body bent forward so as to lengthen the course of the (sciatic) nerve at the hip and knee joints. If the finger is then pressed into the popliteal space so as to make the nerve a little more tense, pain is felt in the course of the nerve at the back of the thigh or above the sciatic notch and behind the hip." A positive test suggests the presence of radiculopathy.

Well-Leg Raising Test (Crossed-Leg Sign):   This test was described by Fayersztajn in 1901. The straight leg raising test is performed on the unaffected limb. In a positive test, contralateral limb pain is produced by such a maneuver.

Femoral Nerve Traction Test: This test is performed with the patient lying on one side. The dependent limb is flexed at the hip and knee. The head is also flexed to increase traction on the cauda equina. The relaxed uppermost lower limb is first maximally extended at the hip and then flexed at the knee. The test is positive when pain radiates down the anterior thigh of that limb. It is a traction test for midlumbar radiculopathies. As in the well-leg raising test, femoral nerve traction on the painless limb may produce contralateral anterior thigh pain.

Fibrositis: Inflammatory change in the fibrous layers investing the trunk musculature, producing local pain and tenderness.

Intermittent Claudication: Periodic limping in response to pain.

Lumbalgia (Lumbago): Low back pain with or without radiation into the buttock and posterior thigh.

Motor Point: A local region within a muscle at which the motor nerve provides innervation.

Piriformis Syndrome: Pain in the buttock and down the limb from sciatic nerve irritation by a spasm or contracture in the piriformis muscle.

Pain, Dermatomal: Pain experienced along the cutaneous distribution of a spinal nerve in a limb.

Pain, Sclerotomal (Referred Pain): Pain experienced in a region that shares a common embryologic origin with the region that is diseased.

Sciatica: Pain along the course of the sciatic nerve.

Thoracic Outlet Syndrome: Neuromuscular dysfunction in the upper limb arising from compression of the subclavian vessels and/or the brachial plexus at the base of the neck.

Trigger Point: A localized area of pain or tenderness that reproduces pain symptoms on application of mechanical pressure and that results from referred pain.

Vertebral Artery Syndrome: Symptoms and signs of muscular inadequacy in the posterior cranial circulation from spondylotic compromise of the vertebral artery.

SURGICAL TERMS

Laminotomy: Creating an opening in one lamina or more.

Laminectomy: Removal of a lamina from its superior to its inferior margin.

Hemilaminectomy: Removal of one half of a lamina.

Bilaminectomy: Removal of two laminae.

Facetectomy: Excision of the articular process that contains the facets of a zygapophyseal joint.

Foraminotomy: Removal of a portion of the wall of the intervertebral foramen.

Pediculectomy: Pedicle excision.

Neural Arch Excision: Self-explanatory.

Spinous Process Excision: Self-explanatory.

Ligamentus Flavum Excision: Self-explanatory.

Transverse Process Excision: Self-explanatory.

Discectomy: Excision of the intervertebral disc, all or part.

Rhizotomy: Surgical transection of a nerve root.

Neurolysis: Separation of a nerve from adhering scar tissue.

Fusion: Anterior Interbody Fusion: Arthrodesis of two or more vertebrae performed by excision of the intervertebral disc and cartilage end-plates and insertion of bone graft between the two vertebrae.

Lateral Fusion: Arthrodesis of two or more vertebrae performed by decorticating and bone grafting the lateral surface of the zygapophyseal joint, the pars interarticularis, and the transverse process, either unilaterally or bilaterally.

Posterior Fusion: Arthrodesis of two or more vertebrae performed by decortication and bone grafting of the neural arches between the right and left zygapophyseal joints.

Posterolateral Fusion: Arthrodesis of two or more vertebrae performed by decorticating and bone grafting the zygapophyseal joint, the pars interarticularis, and the transverse processes, either unilaterally or bilaterally.

Posterior Interbody Fusion: Arthrodesis of two or more vertebrae performed by excising the intervertebral disc through the spinal canal and inserting bone graft into the intervertebral space by the same route.

Posterior Vertebral Osteotomy: Osteotomy performed through the neural arches of two adjacent vertebrae.

Internal Fixation: The binding together of two or more vertebrae with implants of metal or other material.

Facet Rhizotomy (Percutaneous Facet Rhizotomy, Facet Rhizolysis):   Denervation of a zygapophyseal joint by destruction of capsular and pericapsular tissue.

Discography: The introduction of radiopaque fluid into the nucleus pulposus for purposes of identifying disc configuration.

Spinal Nerve-Root: Those neural structures (motor nerve and sensory root) that combine to form a single entity that begins at the emergence from the dura and extends to the level of the sensory ganglion and are invested by an extension of the common dural sac.

INDEX ▬▬▬▬▬▬▬▬

Page numbers in italics represent illustrations. Page numbers followed by t indicate tables.